THE COACH AND US

THE COACH AND US

The True Story of
the Birth
of Holistic Basketball

Norman Kozak
Nathan Yellen

Preface by Ray Meyer

Rutledge Books, Inc.

Danbury, CT

Rutledge Books, Inc.
107 Mill Plain Road, Danbury, CT 06811
1-800-278-8533

Manufactured in the United States of America

Cataloging in Publication Data
Kozak, Norman and Yellen, Nathan
   The coach and us

DEDICATION

*T*his work is dedicated to God and is for all who seek to honor Him by developing their full potential, "doing with all their might whatsoever their hands findeth to do."

All we need to guide us is:

Love,
Think,
DO!

Enter here, all ye who have a passion for truth.

CONTENTS

Preface by Ray Meyer ix
Introduction xi

1. What is Holism? 1
2. The Nature of Holistic Sport and Living. 5
3. Story of The Coach and Us. 13
4. Epilogue: Retirement? 149

About the Authors. 159
Glossary 160
Bibliography 161

ACKNOWLEDGMENT

We deeply express our indebtedness and gratitude to Ray Meyer, "The Coach", whose humility and humanity made possible the events that are the source of this work.

PREFACE

Scripture is filled with proverbs and stories of people who have used faith in God and one's self to accomplish difficult goals. But who among us uses faith at the very highest levels? True happiness follows those who do, for they are in sync with God, humanity, and themselves.

As a coach and as a person, I have tried to instill in my players characteristics that would give them confidence in themselves. I wanted them to be real people. I wanted them to perform at their very best, to be *victors*, not just winners. Sometimes I was successful, other times I was not. I tried using my faith in God and myself to create teams with a capital "T" and real people with a capital "P".

The Coach and Us is not just a basketball story. It is the story of a coach and a group of talented young players who found each other and a "way of living" during the 1983-4 DePaul Basketball Season. It is the story of learning the lessons that can help each of us face life and its problems with the faith, hope, and love that power us forward to do what we must do.

This was my team, as they were all my teams. I hope that you enjoy this book and that it helps your life too.

Ray Meyer

INTRODUCTION

Imagine what competitive sports could be if God were the interface between one team and another; if the human will and the Divine Will were wedded together with such "spiritual voltage" and momentum to enable an athlete to "draw out everything within"; if peak experiences and performances were the rule rather than the exception. That's real performance and great entertainment.

Imagine the reaction, participation and enthusiasm, the thrills and excitement of player and fan, and the glory of God watching a "teamy" team, fully alive, reaching its maximum potential—doing whatever it takes to be victorious.

In the hope of fulfilling all of the above, understanding and love did obtain and an age-old concept with a new twist was expanded to an area heretofore ignored: the birth of Holistic Basketball.

A message for our readers: This book consists of four parts. Part 1 explains holism as we understand it. Part 2 emphasizes holism as a dynamic concept in relation to sport and life; something you do! In Part 3, "Story of the Coach and Us", the main idea advanced is that the impact of "working holism", to a degree, contributed to the success of DePaul during the 1983-84 Basketball Season. "The Coach", Ray

Meyer, served as a holistic model for imitation and the team instinctively capitalized on the information he obtained from us, working uniquely through him, but (as far as we know) never directly communicated to the players. Readers may prefer to start with Part 3 and refer to Parts 1 and 2 for further clarification and enlightenment and to guard against errors in understanding. Part 4 reflects our relationship with Coach after his final game.

It is our sincere wish that this book helps you find spiritual meaning and fulfillment.

1
WHAT IS HOLISM?

The majority of people who are familiar with the concept "holism", probably associate it with holistic medicine. A holistic practitioner treats the WHOLE PERSON, not just the medical problem the patient brings with him. The patient is exhorted to assume responsibility for his own well-being while cooperating with those in whom his health care is entrusted. With this approach, he is not only "taken care of", but "cared about", in the sense that the illness and the total person with the condition are considered.

A holistic practitioner strives to make the individual whole in body, mind, and spirit. When these three dimensions are "properly in tune", so is his relationship to the outside world.

"Wholeness is what we desire most deeply even if we do not know what it is we are striving after and cannot put a name to it...It is also something that encompasses our entire lifetime...It is not something we achieve once and for all. It is not static, a state of being that can be arrived at" (Stein, 1996).

Treating a patient as a whole person represents, in Western Civilization, a rebirth of healing principles that go back in time to Hippocrates, the Greek physician. But the term holistic, "whole", from the Greek "holos", was first coined in 1926 by Jan Christiaan Smuts (1870-1950) in his book, *Holism and Evolution*.

The fundamental principle of the holistic approach is that the whole is more than the sum of its parts. "Just like an automobile is more than just a bunch of nuts and bolts and screws put together, when it comes together it becomes an automobile, which is more than these pieces separately" (Shostrom, 1976); "To a human who watched a movie—instead of seeing a series of still pictures (the separate frames of the film), the viewer would see a continuous "moving image:" (Wittig, 1977).

Going hand in hand with holism is "synergy". To Ruth Benedict (1887-1948), the famous anthropologist, goes the credit as creator of this word. Her use of the term signified the positive "working together" aspect of life in which the combined actions of people will accomplish much more than those who do not work in a spirit of unity.

In societies high in synergy, according to Benedict, the interests of the individual and the interests of the society were identical and mutually reinforcing—the advantage of one being the advantage of the other—and in societies low in synergy there was conflict: the *advantage* of the individual resulted in the *disadvantage* to the group. This indicates the value of a cohesive society in which people work for the good of the whole as they work for the good of themselves: both (the individual and society) are winners.

Those who have built upon Benedict's findings are using her concept of synergy in different systems, with a focus on the parts working together in the service of a common goal, each enhancing and increasing the effectiveness of the others.

Moving forward and upward, in this book our concept of synergy embraces *The American College Encyclopedic Dictionary* definition of synergism: "The doctrine that the human will cooperates with the divine spirit in the work of regeneration." We interpret synergism to mean "Godly holism". Unfortunately, when holism is distinguished in a narrower sense, spirit loses the divine quality it has when synergism dominates, and turns into striving after meaning with God left out. Thus, holism has two faces: the first (religious faith-in-action) does justice to the *whole* of life; the second fails to do so. Consequently, one can be holistic without being synergistic. However, one can't be synergistic without being holistic.

THE NATURE OF HOLISTIC
SPORT AND LIVING

Our philosophy and psychology of holistic sport and living is based upon "becoming a complete person", that is, integrating body, mind, and spirit, through the goal setting and achieving of will, namely, "the capacity to make and implement choices" (Arieti, 1972). Spirit is a fragment of the Divine, the be-all and end-all of life. Rollo May couldn't have been more accurate when he wrote: "Man's task is to unite love and will" (1969). Put slightly differently, Frank Goble affirmed, "the final and highest dimension of will is the development of its spiritual dimension" (1977).

Picture this: A triangle enclosed in a circle with all of its points bordering on the circumference. At the triangle's base, the mind is in one corner and the body in the other; the spiritual dimension is at its apex or midpoint. The circle's circumference symbolizes the "oneness" of the person, resulting when the three levels are functioning in unison.

Ordinarily, the person is orchestrated by the mind governing the body with the spirit playing "second fiddle", but with a change in the direction of the will, a wholesome transforming of the character of a human being takes place. Love becomes the cause, content, and goal of action. The total being becomes spirit-led and motivated; and the mind and body do its bidding. As Copernicus, the celebrated astronomer, disposed of the popular earth-centered theory of the universe in his actual solar-centered system, and exchanged the positions of earth and sun, we interchange the body/mind and spirit, and the spirit becomes the pilot of the person. To borrow a line by the humanistic psychologist, Abraham Maslow, from the context of his theory of human motivation: "...It is as if we have been going north and are now going south instead" (1968).

A *total* commitment to *consciously* internalizing and *living* this new mind-set at all times sets the stage for peak performances, the quintessence in sport and life. Thus, as Lao-Tse, the Chinese philosopher put it, "...love is victorious in attack and invulnerable in defense"; and the more love, the more ability to do! "The most effective and accessible way to acquire the maximum of constructive power is by loving truly and wisely" (Otto, 1972).

So, why not have ALL of ourselves participating in EVERYTHING we do? If a player isn't holistic, then, in a sense, he's not "all there" (pun intended). He's short-changing himself and using a fraction of his productive powers. Doesn't a FRACTION of a person imply a WHOLE to which he originally belonged, from which he is now separated, but ought to reflect and serve, as Spinoza said, "under the aspect of eternity"?

So far we have mentioned the human will, with decision-making as part of its nature, and affirmed the development of spiritual nature as its highest aspect. Will, like spirit, is a sleeping giant and its essence is goal selection and accomplishment. When Emerson wrote, "Nothing great was ever achieved without enthusiasm," he should have included will. Among the powers of the mind, Descartes, the French philosopher, regarded the will as preeminent. It has been called "the man himself" since it is the self's core. No will, no self!

Roberto Assagioli, the psychiatrist, repeatedly emphasized the importance of arousing, awakening, invigorating, and developing the will (1973). Apropos of sports, we hear of the word "intensity". Coaches and writers inquire about a player's intensity, when they really mean his "intensity of will". The level of a player's intensity depends on how strong-willed he is. Intensity, rather than being an explanation, is what needs to be explained, and will is at the root and basis of it! Without the resolution to do, intensity means very little.

It's often been said, "Where there's a will there's a way." The late Green Bay Packers coach, Vince Lombardi, stated: "The difference between a successful person and others is not a lack of strength, not a lack of knowledge, but rather in a lack of will" (Montante, 1991).

As with spirit, will is God-given, awaiting and imploring us to tap this wellspring of power. Just the awareness of will provides an impetus of its own to cultivate it. But we wish to energize the will with more burning desire and force than is necessary for *victory*, for skillful use of will is as exhilarating as *victory*.

To attain this goal, a chief enemy to combat is a player's own resistance to training and developing his will. In many instances, the simple truth or fact is that the player is not willing to make the effort. It takes guts and persistence to overcome ruts and resistance, but ever-present and LASTING motives have to be found to train the will, not only to be powerful and good, but to develop qualities that make it skillful in action. And the best and strongest motive is God's will (Love).

A skillful will is a disciplined will—"no skill without drill!" It "accomplishes more and often does less," time and time again in no time.

According to William James, philosopher/psychologist, "Effort of attention is...the essential phenomenon of will" (1950). For Paul Tillich, it is courage. "Courage," he writes, "listens to reason and carries out the intention of mind" (1952). Calvin Coolidge's view underscores the importance of persistence. He insists,

Nothing in the world can take the place of persistence.

Talent will not;...Genius will not;...Education will not;...Persistence and determination are omnipotent.

In keeping with this, Benjamin Franklin maintains, "He

that can have patience," (a form of persistence) "can have what he will."

In his book, *The Act of Will*, Assagioli elaborates on the technique of "Acting As If" as an application of the skillful will. Sometimes referred to as "acting as though," he says, "this technique consists in acting as if one actually possessed the desired inner state." It makes use of the subjective future to change the present. If an athlete acts "as if" he is the best at his position, he may, with performance become so. This inner game of "assuming a virtue though you have it not," is not "phoniness", but "genuine pretense". Transforming "as if" into reality helps overcome the opponent from within— negative self-talk; all the things we say to ourselves that do us in: "I just can't get myself up for practice," or "I couldn't make a free throw if my life depended on it." Such internal communications can become self-fulfilling prophecies, spawning "hang-ups"—mental "tunnel vision," inferiority complexes, distorted self-images, and self-defeating behavior—that keep us from achievement of goals, unless these harmful self-statements are turned off at WILL and replaced by more expansive, positive, and accurate self-talk.

Creative visualization appears to be a variation of this same theme. "When you visualize, you form vivid pictures in your conscious mind. Then, you continue to keep these pictures of your goals or objectives alive until they sink into your subconscious mind" (Mays, 1991).

While physical effort is part and parcel of acting "as if",

visualization involves primarily mental practice and rehearsal in preparation for the time to perform. During the actual game, the athlete feels confident he can overcome any challenge he faces, having already practiced "all the right moves" perfectly in his mind.

Dr. D.T. Jaffe reported: "One study revealed that athletes who practiced shooting baskets merely by imagining the ball going smoothly into the basket improved as much as those who practiced with a real ball and basket" (1980). And golf professional Jim Colbert contended "...the best performance is invariably preceded by a 'visual picture' of the desired action. Systematically visualizing each shot beforehand helps you establish the desired pattern" (Golf Magazine, 1975). Is there a successful golfer around who does not use this method?

If an athlete focuses his efforts on "winning" or results instead of the task at hand, his level of performance will go down. Dyer (1992) wrote, 'Become detached from the outcome of your actions and paradoxically your level of performance will climb."

Holistic creativity calls for a consciousness in which the unconscious dominates. According to Humphrey's Law, "Once performance of a task has become automatized, conscious thought about the task while performing it impairs performance" (Sutherland, 1989).

Tim McCarver, baseball analyst and former major league player, put it well. He said, "The mind is a great thing as long as you don't have to use it" (Plimpton, 1995). And Yogi Berra, who was a star catcher for the New York Yankees before he was elected to the National Baseball Hall of Fame, said that he couldn't hit and think at the same time.

Self-consciousness (neurotic preoccupation with self) triggers and maintains anxiety which is extinguished to the extent that one focuses on the non-self—"where the action is," that's "where one's head is at!"; while the OPTIMAL amount of resourceful inner-directedness and ego-involvement corrects errors "on the go". Creative disequilibrium, being "keyed up", not "uptight", is what achieves excellence. We agree and close with the opinion of Robert M. Nideffer in his book, "The Inner Athlete" "Obviously, the ideal solution is for an athlete to have an awareness of arousal but to be capable of not letting it result in anxiety—in other words, not being disturbed by worrisome thoughts and feelings" (1976).

3
Story Of The Coach And Us

REMARKS ON THE WRITINGS BETWEEN COACH AND US

The writings in this book are to be read in the light of the circumstances existing at the time they were written. Most of the writings are presented in their original text. With the others, information has been omitted, added, and modified without changing their basic form, where we felt simplification and clarification were necessary.

This story began with a series of "off-the-cuff" telephone conversations between Us, Nate, a DePaul alumnus, and Norm, a University of Illinois graduate and close friend of Nate. Below is a concise synopsis of our remarks.

Nate: Norm, are you watching the DePaul game?

Norm: Yeah, it looks like they're (Blue Demons) goin' to luck out again, although you and I both know things aren't right while they're winning.

Nate: M-hm. (Short pause) Uh, it seems their "game plan" doesn't last the full forty minutes. Remember how they played against Larry Bird and Indiana State in the Final Four. That was a nip and tuck affair played to the limits of mental and physical performance...Knew that the excellence displayed by the Demons displaced despair even though they were defeated!

Norm: Yes, the players and the team sure could hold their heads   high, for they were defeated with honor; but now they need to get with it—they don't seem to have their act together—at least not consistently.

Nate: (Laughs) You're right.

Norm: (Concerned) You know what DePaul needs, I mean,—I think the school ought to play Holistic Basketball.

Nate: You know, I've heard of that word (holistic) before. Uh, what does it mean?

Norm: Oh, regarding human behavior, to me, it means the spiritual nature of the person is the driving force and the body and personality or mind are cooperating with it all at once; yet, in a nutshell, if all three dimensions aren't taken into account—with the spirit "runnin' the show"—well, then, the person is incomplete, but when they're in sync, then we have a situation where there's a whole lot more than meets the eye.

Nate: I see. Sounds interesting.

Norm: It's like Emerson said, "Give All to Love." Love is, if not undeveloped, one of the most underdeveloped human resources, and..."perhaps the most powerful form of energy" (Keck, 1978); so why not exploit its capacity to the fullest? I'm sure humankind would have a lot more "peak experiences" if they would.

Nate: M-hm. But you're not only talking about basketball. This pertains to everything in life.

Norm: Exactly. It doesn't matter whether you're playing tiddly winks, hanging wallpaper, or whatever.

Nate: (Thinking) Could we say that "winning holistically" would really be VICTORY, and "losing holistically" could be called DEFEAT?

Norm: Precisely! And the opposite also obtains. By itself, "winning" would be ignominious or disgraceful winning and "losing" would be losing by default or sloppy play.

Nate: You make it sound like teams that are evenly matched in talent—like the team "fired up holistically" would make "duck soup" of the other—be a shoo-in!

Norm: You betcha—and in short order!

Nate: So, by holistic effort we seek the conclusiveness of VIC-TORY, and if that is not possible, honorable DEFEAT, which in reality, except for the score, is the same.

Norm: Yeah. That's right.

Nate: Sure sounds like a Godly way of doing things.

Norm: The only way!..."Man at his best is like God" (Hordern, 1955).

Nate: You know, I, I (stuttering) think I'll call Coach Ray Meyer (DePaul) and see if we can talk to him about this.

Norm: Are you kidding? He probably won't listen to us.

Nate: If any coach will, he will. He's got a lot of character. Will you go with me if I can make an appointment with him?

Norm: Sure!

March 25, 1979

Coach Ray Meyer
DePaul University
Chicago, Illinois

Dear Ray:

I saw and recorded the Final Four game in which Indiana State came out with a 76-74 win over DePaul, but it was no victory in spite of the great game that they played. I just had to write you and thank you for such a fine performance. An editorial that WBBM aired recently (John Madigan, copy enclosed) echoes my sentiments. This game will be remembered almost in its entirety as one of the finest examples of "purist" basketball ever seen, with the full coordination of the mental and physical capabilities of both teams performing at their best—and THAT is what counts! Winning or losing is not really part of the equation. I learned that as a kid, indirectly from you, because your philosophy guided the coaches who guided us: press on their end, run on our end. Never quit. Always do what you have to DO!

There were no losers in this game. It was first class all the way. I think this game will be remembered, not as the game Indiana State won, but as the game DePaul failed to win. Larry Bird and his teammates played extraordinarily well.

Indiana State should have won this game by at least 15-20 points. They played as close to perfection as anyone will ever see. They outlasted us but they did not annihilate us. We were victorious even in defeat and they knew it. Coach, there is a message to be learned from this game and you expressed it on National TV. Summing up the game, you said: "Basketball is a game of mistakes even in a very good game with two fine teams. We made one more (mistake) than they did."

I recall at the end of another game with UCLA, when with about a 14 point lead, we tried a full-court pass and overthrew the ball. The momentum shifted to UCLA and you could feel it. The whittling away of DePaul's lead was assured, but how would the team rise to stem UCLA's charge? That is where quality and "professionalism" shows—in the ability to reach down and find whatever it takes to DO the job. This is what I choose to remember about you and the team. You bring honor to the name Coach!

Cordially,
Nathan Yellen

WBBM NEWSRAD))I(() 78

JOHN MADIGAN NEWS AND COMMENTARY
Tuesday, March 20, 1979

Neither Leo Durocher nor Vince Lombardi were probably as insanely attached to victory as might be indicated by those notorious expressions attributed to them.

And despite the excesses of George Patton and Woody Hayes under stressful moments they surely had to have a reasonable scale of values to attain lasting success.

Even Ray Meyer...according to people who know him best...such as DePaul President, John Cortelyou...of ballplayers, to whom he gave the HIP in high school or college...will tell you Meyer could and can be explosive.

Let no one think...now that Meyer has become sort of a 65-year-old folk hero to Mormons and Catholics...and a lot of other persuasions in between...that he is a walking St. Francis of Assisi.

He always has and does stand up for his rights...and can blow his temper at referees or coaches or players when he thinks the cause is just. But...as Father Cortelyou...who has had a close relationship with him for 38 years...can tell you:

"Ray is never vicious or out-of-control. He'll blow up. But he'll always listen to reason. He's always a gentleman at the core." So it is refreshing in these closing days of what is always one of the most exciting sports periods in the year...the finals of the NCAA Basketball Championship...that someone like Ray Meyer has won the hearts of sports fans everywhere.

Many of whom never heard of DePaul. But now have made sentimental favorite of that paunchy...gray-haired man...with the open-tooth smile who...as Al McGuire said on National TV...took over St. Patricks' Day without even being Irish.

Strong...muscular...outsized athletes...drawing outsized salaries...get all the attention in all the sports these days. Doing sometimes heroic but sometimes zany and irresponsible things...on and off the field.

But for a few days at least...and in areas far beyond Chicago...a rumpled poor-boy-type...sitting on the sidelines...who has won more games than any other active basketball coach...is everybody's lovable Dutch Uncle.

Nice guys don't have to finish last. It just takes them a little longer...when they don't think winning is the only thing in life.

John Madigan WBBM Newsradio 78
January 31, 1981

January 31, 1981

Ray Meyer, Coach
DePaul University
Chicago, Illinois

Dear Coach:

While viewing the Syracuse game, I realized that there is a problem on the floor that doesn't show up in your "good" practice sessions—where indeed the games are won! You called it last week during a TV interview, and the despair in your voice was noticeable. Not defeat, but frustration. You've got the soldiers, but they seemed to be blowing the battle! Coach, a friend and I think that something has been lost in your communication with them.

Everyone knows you have the goods and the boys have the stuff, but they are not doing it consistently. They have it in them to be like the Chicago Symphony Orchestra (the only other quality team in Chicago besides DePaul)—poetry in motion as they played in the second half of the Syracuse game. That's what they are all about and while I don't expect performance like that all the time—it sure was nice! They had gotten beyond the first-half control game of Syracuse—as a *team*. Perhaps that is it: they were a team, not individuals as you said. You have to find out why they don't play as a team for the entire game. Communicate!

I hope this is helpful to you and the team. Please note the article in Monday's Sun-Times; it surely gets to the core. They (the players) are "punishing" you for something. They give you what you want in practice, and play as they want in the game. We are DePaul!

Nathan Yellen

DePaul University

Department of Athletics	1011 West Belden Avenue Chicago, IL 60614	312/321-8010

February 4, 1981

Mr. Nathan Yellen
7327 North Kedvale Avenue
Lincolnwood, IL 60646

Dear Nathan:

I want to thank you for taking the time to write and express
your views.

There are a few problems behind the scenes which cannot be
aired. These have to be resolved before we can become a great
team. We are making great strides eliminating them. The
chemistry is not right at this time; however, the players are
aware of it, and they are working very hard to get things flow-
ing smoothly. I look forward to improvement with each game
from now on.

With best wishes and kindest personal regards, I am,

Yours,
Ray Meyer
Head Basketball Coach

For the 1979-80, '80-81, and '81-82 basketball seasons, DePaul amassed an unmatched record of regular season winning percentages; yet the media downplayed the team's record and achievements after DePaul was disappointing in NCAA (National Collegiate Athletic Association) tournament play. Coach's critics focused on the part and ignored the whole.

Before the '82 tourney began, DePaul played an exhibition game against Athletes In Action, a God-devoted team comprised of former high school and college players who enjoy the game and provide more than just interesting scrimmages for college basketball teams. Mind you, DePaul was ranked No. 2 in the nation on March 5, 1982, with a record of 26-1 when Athletes In Action proceeded to beat the Blue Demons 91-86. This AIA team used the power of GOD to marshal its forces against DePaul, and we learned something that night that would change forever our concept of how this game must be played. By God, we DID learn!

We learned how empowering religious faith-in-action is. It makes things happen that would not happen without it.

Nine days after the loss to AIA, the 1981-82 Basketball Season for DePaul ended on a sad note. After leading 8-0, the team lost to Boston College 85-72. For the third year in a row, DePaul failed to get past its first game in NCAA tournament play.

March 28, 1982

Coach Ray Meyer
Assistant Coach Joey Meyer
DePaul University
Chicago, Illinois

Dear Coaches:

The 1982-83 season began for us eight minutes into the Boston College game—for WE *ARE* DePaul, *all* of us. I have carefully watched our team these past four years and made some observations of significance, some stemming back that far, culminating in my letter (Jan. 31, 1981) answered by Coach (Feb. 4, 1981—copy enclosed). It is my earnest desire to share these thoughts with you, for they are of great relevance to the team and you at this time, and well into the future.

I assure you that my thoughts are considered and of great applicability. If you would give me 45 minutes to relate them, I believe you would agree. Please grant me this time now.

Yours in DePaul,
Nathan Yellen

DePaul University

Department of Athletics   1011 West Belden Avenue   312/321-8010
                                 Chicago, IL 60614

Dear Nathan,

I read your letter and your request for time to talk about some thoughts of yours.

For the next two weeks, I will be very busy answering the mail. I suggest you call me and we will make a date.

Yours,

Ray Meyer

Our first personal contact with Coach was on April 27, 1982. We met him in his private office at DePaul University. He welcomed us in his characteristic, unassuming manner, wondering what our purpose was in coming to see him. He was very relaxed and we felt very comfortable in his presence.

After exchanging pleasantries, we introduced and explained the holistic approach to Coach. We left with him our writing "HOLISTIC BASKETBALL", our "game plan" that deals with creativity as a function of the participation of the *total* person. We also brought a book along called *Holistic Running*, which Coach asked us if he could read. He thanked us for the book.

The 50 minutes we shared with Coach—a real eye-opener to Coach—seemed like 5!

HOLISTIC BASKETBALL

Congratulations, Coach, and good luck for the 1982-83 season. I'd like to introduce my friend, Norm Kozak, and myself, Nate Yellen. We want to thank you for taking the time to give us an opportunity to express ourselves on the subject of holism. Holism would say "Good Luck—but the less you need, the better!"

Holism, as you can see from the books that we've brought along today, has been extended to an ever increasing array of subjects. In front of us we can see that it has been directly applied to running, the treatment of headaches and learning disorders, the social sciences and of course, classically, to the field of medicine with the various "Gestalt" theories and applications that have grown up, such as Positive Mental Attitude (PMA) and the revival of Zen Buddhism and the like, attempting to deal with the problems relating to the integration of mind and body.

We will start then by saying that holism is the theory of "wholes" or totals which are *more* than the sum of their parts. There are jigsaw puzzles that are comprised of many parts that convey nothing, until put together; then they portray a beautiful picture. We also have animated cartoons that are a series of still pictures flashed in front of a camera giving the feeling or the appearance of movement and animation, but that are still pictures, nonetheless. What about the athlete who seems to be driving himself to produce at a rate of 150 percent, doing more than appears to other people's eyes to be possible? There are endless instances that we could cite, but these examples show us that wholes cannot be reduced to any part or all parts. The parts do not function in isolation but as parts of a whole, and must be considered as such.

Going along with holism is "synergism". Synergism links the human will with the divine spirit; thereby the whole of human behavior becomes more than the sum of its parts.

The word "holism" was first introduced by Jan Christiaan Smuts (1870-1950), the South African soldier/statesman, who wrote extensively on this subject over 60 years ago in his book *Holism and Evolution*. He strove in his lifetime toward unity, being one of the early leaders of the League of Nations. Prior to him, in the 12th century, Moses Maimonides (1135-1204) was also a believer in holistic principles, having clearly used them in his profession as a doctor, a rabbi, and a philosopher in the Aristotelian method. A noted doctor, Maimonides treated the whole being—body, mind, and spirit—of the patient, while dedicating his whole being to God.

The greatness of Maimonides and his difference between the eminent Greek physician, Galen, has been expressed in the following poem:

> *Galen's art heals only the body,*
> *Maimon's the flesh and spirit both.*
> *Just as his knowledge has made him the physician of the century,*

So too he heals the disease of ignorance with wisdom.
The moon entrusts itself to his art,
He heals it of the infirmities that sometimes afflict it,
The spots in the time of the full moon
And the pain of the moon's waning (Heschel, 1982).

Coach, over the years, we have unknowingly applied holistic concepts to our lives, as you and many others have, too, some by design and/or by chance. Now, in these times we are explicitly aware, as these books tell us, that the scientific application of holistic principles brings greater productivity. In our opinion, the holistic method can and should be applied to basketball as it was applied to the sport of running. Both sports condition the whole person to act under control and without compulsion.

What is Holistic Basketball? It is an approach to basketball that deals with the whole being of each player. Along with a player's physical abilities, it focuses on his mental and spiritual development. This approach, while viewing the player as a unified whole, takes all three dimensions into account. It emphasizes that the player see himself as a whole, yet part of a larger whole—the team. Of necessity, the holistic viewpoint treats the player as an end in himself, never only as a means. It asks the player what he's experiencing, while observing his behavior and play. It uses this knowledge to help the player help himself and the team. This holistic method gives special consideration to the player's "way of living". It helps him choose a meaningful direction-giving goal and implements a plan for its realization.

When a player "gives his all", the chances are good his total effort will rub off on every player. If it does, the totality of the team's efforts will become more than the sum of each player's effort considered separately. Consequently, the whole team will attain the goal it desires.

We do not mean to say that the "holistic way" is a substitute for talent or creates it. It draws out talent that is impeded or blocked and builds on it. As the player begins to play for the better, the team becomes better.

Coach, here are six tips to start your holistic program rolling. You can:

1. Continue to ask God for guidance.
2. Be open-minded.
3. Reach each player even before he enters school, and provide him with all the holistic information and materials that can really be helpful: films, tapes, books, literature, visual aids, etc.
4. Arouse, awaken, and develop within each player the desire, if needed, to excel. If he has the desire, then help him to increase it so that he inspires all other players to excel at their highest and enjoy the holistic/synergistic experience.
5. Teach each player to become self-dependent, to be his own source of drive and energy.

6. Clear up "fuzzy" thinking. "Telling it like it is", with love, changes fundamental misconceptions and fosters clarity of thought which shapes action. "Where the soul is pure, the thought is clear," says the proverb. And clear-headedness erases and prevents compulsive and disorganized behavior. Holism and compulsion are opposites! Easy does it—that's the holistic way!

To repeat: In our opinion, holistic thought as employed successfully in medicine, running, the social sciences, etc., can and should be extended to basketball. This would enable the whole team to perform maximally and achieve its goal. Frustrating this achievement can be one or more players who have not been reached holistically, affecting the other teammates and causing the whole team to play below its potential.

There is no team (that we know of) that has the "know-how" to apply holism to basketball; and how many of these teams that may be familiar with holistic principles have researched them in depth?

Thanks once again for your time and we hope you can understand why we said "Good Luck" in our opening. We also said "the less you need, the better!" Good Luck is what we wish the opposing team. We prefer "working holism".

Remember, we welcome your questions. We are DePaul.

April 27, 1982

April 30, 1982

Dear Coach:

I can't recall when I've spent a more enjoyable 50 minutes in a very long time! Aware that, on such little sleep and a grueling schedule, you met with us, listened and joined into our talk on holism, is more than Norm and I could expect; but you gave it to us. That is holism in action—the 150 percent of life! Thanks—I hope you found useful and enjoyable *Holistic Running*.

If you are interested in pursuing further the discussion elevated to practical applications, we are willing and waiting to learn of the new dawn of B-Ball!

Warm regards,
Nathan Yellen

DePaul University

| Department of Athletics | 1011 West Belden Avenue
Chicago, IL 60614 | 312/321-8010 |

May 25, 1982

Dear Nate:

I have finished *Holistic Running* and found it very interesting and enlightening. In fact, I read a few of the chapters several times.

There is a lot to be learned from this approach to athletics. I am thinking and figuring ways I may join some of the thoughts to basketball. We want our players relaxed and happy in their practices and games. They will get more out of their activities and I will get more basketball out of them.

Nate, you may stop by any time for the book and I will talk to you as long as I can.

> Yours,
> Ray Meyer

May 26, 1982

Dear Coach:

I am so pleased to learn that you enjoyed *Holistic Running*, and found it, as you said, "interesting and enlightening." Your note is proof of your acceptance of the applicability of holism to basketball: "Thinking, learning, applying, and doing!" I have just finished A.J. Heschel's *Maimonides* (biography) and it knocked me for a loop; all the phrases and "the" master plan—Meaning, Accomplishment, and Direction; it's awesome. The book is a spiritual odyssey—striving after wholeness with all life and God. Exciting indeed! I'll be by for it soon—the book. Be well!

Warmest regards
Nate

In the introduction to *Holistic Running* by Joel Henning, the editor of the magazine The Jogger, Bernard L. Gladieux, Jr., writes: "For Joel Henning and perhaps millions of others, running is as much a mental and spiritual experience as it is an exquisitely physical pastime. The integration of the whole person—body, mind, and soul—in the activity of running can be a mystical experience."

And in Henning's own words: "The overwhelming majority of runners have little need to race in competition at all...Our satisfactions are internal...Our running begins to keep our bodies fit and to satisfy our need for play, but it also progresses through stages of deeper meaning to expand our self-awareness, to become a holistic aspect of our lives. It is indeed a form of worship, an attempt to find God, a means to the transcendent...I have power, power that propels me cross country, puts me intimately in touch with nature, strengthens my body, expands my mind...I own the day...For me, holistic running...continues to help me understand myself and the world...I accomplish more than I ever did before, and I have greater inner strength."

With a further evolution in our thinking, our paper "HOLISTIC BASKETBALL" appeared to us as a "diamond in the rough along the edges". While we feel it is correct, it only skirted the issue of "peak experiences", and never explicitly referred to them. "HOLISTIC INSPIRITING" is our follow-up and improvement upon "HOLISTIC BASKETBALL", and represents a continuing crystallization of our thought.

HOLISTIC INSPIRITING
By
Norm Kozak

My purpose in this writing is to help persons become what they were meant to be, "fully functioning", so that they can enjoy repeated "peak experiences" without the use of mind-changing drugs or alcohol.

Why are "peak experiences" so rare? The answer stems largely from the fact that man's spiritual nature is being ignored. Science disavows the intangible spirit altogether. Science bases its knowledge on observation and experimentation. Since spirit is an invisible power, a gift of faith, science regards it as a metaphysical, mystical concept outside its purview of "hard facts".

"True, my power is invisible," says the spirit. But "only those who can see the invisible can do the impossible"; "you" scientists "see things as they are; and you ask Why?" But I dream things that never were; and I ask "Why not?" And besides, isn't your value-free science itself a value?

If the spirit could speak to the person it would probably say, "I'm down here in the basement of your mind clanging my bells for attention, but you're so busy worshipping the golden calf of material success that you won't even take time to listen. Well, I want to be heard! I am the silent, small voice of God. And I'm silent for a reason! If I were so loud and distinct that I forced myself upon you, I would be denying you freedom of choice. You would be a puppet in the hands of God, but God is no 'divine puppeteer'. He wants you to choose to become what you are and ought to be."

The spirit continues, "In a sense I'm an enemy, but I'm a friendly enemy. I'm the threat to your present 'way of living'. I call your very being into question, and you don't like that, because you'd rather continue your familiar old pattern rather than consider the possibility of changing. In the twilight of life I don't want you feeling as the Peggy Lee song goes, 'Is that all there is?' Rather I want you to have enjoyed what there was and look forward with confidence to what is yet to be! Here and now I want you to sing along with Tom Jones that even though 'I had conquered the world...without love I had nothing at all'; and to learn, just as Nat "King" Cole's "Nature Boy", that "The greatest thing you'll ever learn is just to love and be loved in return."

Inspiriting is the process of awakening, developing, and infusing new spirit or life within the self. It is a journey, not a destination. As John Dewey said, "Not perfection as a final goal but the ever enduring process of perfecting, maturing, refining, is the aim of living." The partial achievement of inspiriting leaves us better off than if we had made no attempt at all.

Inspiriting questions are: "Are we fulfilling our personal needs for security, love and belongingness, and self-esteem?" "How do we work on and express being loving?" "What meaningful goals, purposes, and values shall we pursue?"

"Why not vow to put a soul into our goal?"

Inspiriting is a holistic (whole) process. It deals with all the dimensions of a person—body, mind, and spirit. The body is the physical dimension of a person's being; the mind is the psychological (thinking/willing/feeling) part; spirit is the HOLY inside you.

The body is viewed as a whole in itself and yet part of a larger whole—mind-body. Similarly, mind-body is a whole and part of the total person—spirit-mind-body. None of these parts are conceived in isolation from their context, but rather as aspects of a totality. Moreover, the total person is never abstracted from the physical world and culture of which he is a part.

Holistic Inspiriting aims at recentering the total personality around the spirit or will of God. When body and mind, through the personal will, are guided and directed by the spirit, holistic energies and powers are channeled at their peak, and the whole or total becomes more than the sum of its parts.

Difficulties abound when body and mind operate independently and at cross purposes to the spirit. Anxiety and compulsive behavior result. Self-love is transformed into its very opposite—selfishness. The part has taken control of the whole. The person's lifestyle now resists the spirit's unfolding.

Once a person is *totally* committed to the inspiriting process, the process feeds on itself. Ultimately, as unifying center of the person, the inspiriting process leads to ongoing fulfillment.

BIBLICAL GROUNDS FOR HOLISTIC INSPIRITING

For the sake of clarity and simplicity most of the following biblical passages are identified and paraphrased in contemporary English to illustrate the spiritual applicability of holistic/synergistic behavior:

1. "Make love your aim." (1 Cor. 14:1)
   "Love" is used in the sense of (1) "Love the Lord your God with all your heart and all your soul and all your might," and (2) "Love your neighbor as yourself."
2. "Love covers a multitude of sins." (Prov. 17:9)
3. "Pay all your debts except the love for another. Never finish paying that." (Rom. 13:8)
4. "Love is the fulfillment of the law." (Rom. 13:10)
   "The law is spiritual." (Rom. 7:14)
5. "The written code kills but the spirit gives life." (2 Cor. 3:6)
6. "Not by might nor by power but by my spirit," says the Lord Almighty. (Zech. 4:6)
7. "Be ye transformed by the renewing of your mind." (Rom. 12:2)
8. "With God all things are possible." (Matt. 19:26)
9. "We should make plans counting on God to direct us." (Prov. 16:9)
10. "God always keeps his promises." (Rom. 11:29)
11. "Commit your work to the Lord, then it will succeed." (Prov. 16:3)

12. "See how the Lord God does things, and fall in line. Don't fight the facts of nature." (Eccles. 7:13)

13. "If God is on our side, who can ever be against us." (Rom. 8:31) "Who are you to criticize God?" (Rom. 9:20)

14. "If a kingdom is divided against itself, that kingdom cannot stand." (Mark 3:24)

15. "Pride separates us from God and leads to spiritual deadness." (Prov. 16:18)

16. "It is senseless to pay tuition to educate a rebel who has no heart for truth." (Prov. 17:16)

17. "But the fruit of the Spirit is love, joy, peace, patience, kindness, goodness, faithfulness, gentleness, and self-control." (Gal. 5:22-23)

Then, as fate would have it, there appeared a truly remarkable film entitled *Chariots of Fire*, that showed the practical evidence of the validity of the holistic approach to sport and life. This true story centered on two runners, both of whom looked forward to winning gold medals in the 1924 Paris Olympics, but with different motivations.

One, an Englishman, Harold Abrahams, was driven by vanity, a compulsive search for identity and certainty in order to still his tormenting doubts regarding himself. He maintained, "...If I can't win, I won't run." The other was a Scotsman, Eric Liddell, not a problem to himself, who ran, lived, and performed for God, using his talents to the fullest, in order to better serve Him. "To win is to honor Him," the Scot said.

When this movie is viewed in relation to the holistic information that Coach and we had shared, we see that each reflects the other. Here was not only a manifestation of our thought, but a true, living reaffirmation of it!

We learned from this award-winning picture that the source of VICTORY by design and the healing balm to assuage DEFEAT were identical! Satisfaction with self through holistic performance was EVERYTHING! VICTORY brought no special elation and DEFEAT had no sting; they were the same, for the controlled maximum effort was the release. Performance merged into plan and execution brought the true reward—peace and satisfaction.

What did people really learn from the *Chariots* story,

though they enjoyed it? Very little; we MOVED...as we were MOVED!!! Coach was preparing for his Summer Basketball Camp and we called to tell him of our find.

July 7, 1982

Dear Coach: (At Basketball Camp, 3 Rivers, Wisconsin)

I know that you are in the "Happy Hunting Ground" and further that you have a smile on your face! Enjoy! I have discovered that now there is no videotape of *Chariots of Fire*. You'll have to go see it at the movies yourself. Please view it in as close to a hungry state as you can be and if you find tears appropriate, that's O.K. too. Remember—go see it on an empty stomach. I'll pop for popcorn (no butter). If at the conclusion of the film you wish to speak with someone, I volunteer two ears ANY HOUR—DAY or NIGHT. I have so much to tell you on holism/synergism that will astound you; also a proposal you will be unable to refuse! We have discovered the important thing in life!

Warmest regards,
Nathan Yellen

August 18, 1982

Dear Coach:

I hope you've had a totally rewarding summer camp—one that has prepared you for this fall and winter. Norm and I have thought and spoken of you many times this summer. We hope that you had a chance to see *Chariots of Fire*. We want to see it again.

I would imagine that your first days back next week will be no less than horrendous. You will need special strength to face them. Norm and I pray that God grants you the strength to do *all* that you must do! No more, but certainly no less!

Warmest regards,
Nathan Yellen

September 17, 1982

Dear Coach:

Norm and I just heard of the tragic passing of Bill Robinzine, Jr., (suicide). Please accept our most sincerely extended condolences. His life must have really been something. The story in the newspaper about him probably doesn't even scratch the surface. The walk-on* who made it during those dark days in the fortunes of DePaul: What a heart! It is that, that you must remember in all of this. What he did and how he did it, that's what counts. You must honor his life and not his passing, and strive to prevent such future occurrences. Bear up—you honor him and his life.

What a fitting tribute if this season could be dedicated in his honor and that basketball life that would have been missed, but for his dad and you. The walk-on that made it was a real, whole man! It should have been recognized earlier. Our sincere condolences to his folks and family are also extended.

Warmly,
Norm Kozak
Nate Yellen

* An athlete who tries out for a college team without being recruited.

DePaul University

Department of Athletics   1011 West Belden Avenue   312/321-8010
                                 Chicago, IL 60614

October 4, 1982

Mr. Nathan Yellen
5306 W. Devon Ave.
Chicago, IL 60646

Dear Nate:

Chariots of Fire is a very inspiring film. You have to believe that, with God's help, plus a strong belief in yourself, you really are capable of performing as a champion. You are the best.

As a coach, I subscribe to the thought that state of mind is the key to success in sports. Once you are physically capable of playing, it is up to the mind. An athlete sets goals for himself and they are high. The higher the goal, the more competitive it will be to reach that goal. The more competitive situations will have the strongest motivational effect. Motivation is getting the maximum potential out of an athlete.

Chariots of Fire is a very moving and realistic movie. It is about belief and love. An athlete can do many things if he believes in himself. It is an excellent movie, portraying holism to the greatest degree possible. The athlete believes in himself, and he trains exceptionally hard to be successful. His beliefs give him the aggressiveness, determination, self-confidence, emotional control, and the mental toughness. He (Eric Liddell, the Scotsman who ran and lived to serve God) had the strength and the will to push himself to greater heights than he had ever reached before. His faith drove him.

I am very sorry about Bill Robinzine. I never thought he would do away with himself. I still can't believe it. We are holding a memorial service for him Wednesday night at five o'clock. Also, we are hoping to establish a scholarship in his honor. I loved that guy.

Your film (a videotape of *Chariots of Fire*) was shown to our track and soccer teams for inspirational and motivational purposes.

I wish to thank you again for the assistance and advice you have rendered me.

Sincerely,
Ray Meyer

RM:pb (encl.)

Note: Now, there was no doubt that our five-month association with coach was fruitful, or that he regarded us as true friends. Coach saw "working holism" as a viable resource. But would he pursue it and use it? And, if so, when and how?

Muhammad Ali, the former heavyweight boxing champion of the world, echoed the words Coach expressed on "belief" at the beginning of his October 4 letter. Ali said, "To be a champion you must believe you are the best. If not, pretend you are" (Robbins & McClendon III, 1997). For the word "pretend", we substitute the phrase "play as if". It is our belief that if a player would "play as if" he's the best at his position, maybe he would be. Maybe the whole team would "play as if" too.

For an athlete, "The more competitive situations will have the strongest motivational effect," Coach said in the second paragraph of his letter. A question comes to mind. In competitive situations, should an athlete strive for perfection or excellence? Many motivational authorities (speakers and authors) praise the "pursuit of excellence" and discredit the striving for perfection. These authorities fail to notice the important difference between a healthy striving for perfection and a striving for perfection that is unhealthy.

Striving for perfection is unhealthy when an athlete has unrealistic expectations regarding how he *should* perform. His "inner critic" will constantly berate him if he fails to measure up to his "shoulds", thereby compounding his fear of failure.

Healthy striving for perfection eases an athlete's inner torment and the pressure to perform caused by his "shoulds". Dr. Harold Greenwald, co-author of *The Happy Person*, affirmed: "*Striving* for perfection...can be very useful—if we don't attack ourselves when we don't live up to an impossible demand" (1984). "Phychologist Albert Ellis believes we would be better off if we simply banished the word *should* from our vocabularies. He suggests substituting the expression: "It would be better if..."" (Freeman & DeWolf, 1992).

In brief, the joy of true excellence is achieved as a by-product of the healthy striving for perfection.

Toward the close of the third paragraph in his letter, Coach mentioned the term "mental toughness". What does mental toughness mean? Obviously, it means different things to different people.

On radio station WSCR-AM in Chicago, Illinois, Mike Ditka, National Football League Hall of Famer, defined mental toughness as "the ability to perform at your maximum under the maximum amount of pressure."

Toughness is physical as well as mental. Loehr (1994) said, "Toughness is the ability to consistently perform toward the upper range of your talent and skill regardless of competitive circumstances."

In the DePaul colors of blue and red, a 22 x 34" watercolor print, called "Coach", was made of Coach Ray. Soon the print would be unveiled at a party in Coach's honor at Lake View Bank in Chicago. Funds raised from the sale of the prints would be used to support DePaul athletics. Each print would be numbered and pencil signed by Coach and the artist.

Coach asked Nate for his opinion of the watercolor and referred Nate to the party chairman. When the chairman showed Nate the print, he liked it. He felt it captured the spirit and being of Coach, and told him so. Coach was pleased.

At the party, a photographer took a picture of Coach and us while we were discussing baseball, Coach's second favorite sport. Spending 15 minutes or more talking with Coach was a memorable experience, indeed. We also had the honor of being introduced to Mrs. Meyer.

November 8, 1992

Dear Coach:

Just a line to let you know that Norm and I thought that the unveiling of the picture and the party were a huge success, and we hope that good comes from it. We shall never forget your "chewing the fat" with us over baseball, another facet of Coach Ray Meyer. It's nice to say that you are one fine man in a world where there are few who work at it. Take care and go with God!

Nate

November 15, 1982

Dear Coach:

I had hoped that we would speak once before the season began, and now it's here. Time sure flies. Each day I hope you put in your suit lapel one of the "you are loved" pins Norm and I gave you. The pin is symbolic of what life is all about, and we gave the pins to you from our hearts. Norm and I found our experience with you on holism/synergism most elevating. We are hopeful that we can be of service to you in developing a program of mind-set in this regard. We still believe such a program would improve the response of the team even if only one player is reached. And you know that we have more than just that on our minds.

We could not and would not put on the hard sell for you to get into this kind of program, for such a decision had to be totally voluntary, yours and yours alone. I think that you believe in the idea of a holistic/synergistic approach and hope you are able to use some of the principles to your benefit. In trying to reach you a few days ago, I wanted to say that UCLA is now reviewing (CBS News) its sports program in the light of developing the "total" person, to help him to make the most of himself in sport and life. It is an idea whose time has come. Needless to say—any time, any place is yours if you want to discuss or do something on this subject. You know how strongly we feel about how effective this idea is. It's yours for the asking and it's all up to you. We want you to feel that you can "chew the fat" with us on any other subject as well, and we would be honored to listen and talk back, if you wished.

Enclosed is my ticket and game review of the Athletes In Action game (3/5/82). They are intended for you as a reminder to stay away (as best you can) from the conditions that foster compulsive behavior—the never ending struggle that faces us all.

We also have unsigned "Coach" prints (Numbers 6 & 7) that we would treasure even more if inscribed by you—any time you wish.

Be well, do well, and take care. You are loved. That is the message in all we've said.

Fondest regards,
Nate and Norm

November 25, 1982

Dear Coach:

We just received the photo that was taken of you, Norm, and myself during the unveiling of your watercolor at the Lake View Bank party. Thank you so very much for helping us obtain it. Norm and I shall always treasure it as a memento of you and that special conversation that we shared.

We have spoken much about you and the team in the past two weeks. We are happy to get this season on the road finally, as we are sure you are too. God love you and your endeavor and grant you success. We are DePaul.

Warmest regards,

Nate

December 21, 1982

Dear Coach:

Although we know only you, and we briefly were introduced to Mrs. Meyer (at the party), we feel as though we are at one with you and your family through love of the game and devotion to the spirit that moves us all. We sincerely wish you and your family a very Merry Christmas and a happy, healthy new year that finds your cup filled to the brim by the Almighty with all those things that make life meaningful and fulfilling.

We can wish you nothing better than "A Synergistic 1983" to you and yours, the team, and DePaul in all your undertakings.

Warm regards,
Norm and Nate

A SYNERGISTIC MAN

As a kid growing up on the South Side of Chicago, interested in all sports, it was my (Nate) good fortune to meet a fine gentleman, Jesse Owens. At almost every major sports function where a guest speaker was needed, Jesse was there—Hi-Y, BBYO (B'nai B'rith Youth Organization), Chicago Park District, etc. At the time I wasn't sure what he was famous for, and understood little of the man, but his words ring in my ears today! "If it's worth doing—do it well!" He claimed one should try his hardest, never quit, and always have faith in himself and God. He admitted that he drove himself to go further when it seemed he couldn't go any further. He advised to do good, not to say or do bad.

This humble man always had time for kids, and although he was treated poorly by this nation that he loved and denied the fame and wealth that he so richly deserved, he never stopped giving of himself. He was Mister Drive, Think, and Do! No less. His reward came from helping those who had the honor of knowing him.

His feats are legendary and serve as an example of what a person can do with belief in self, drive, and love of God. He stands as a shining model of all that is good in man. He was tested as a sophomore at Ohio State University, and on May 25, 1935, in a 45 minute time span, he accomplished the following: THE GREATEST 45 MINUTES IN THE PERSONAL

HISTORY OF TRACK AND FIELD EVENTS

3:15 Won the 100 yard dash in 9.4 seconds, tying the world record.

3:25 In one jump, leaped 26 feet, 8 1/4 inches, breaking the world record by six inches.

3:45 Won the 220 yard dash in 20.3 seconds, breaking the world record by 3/10.

4:00 Won the 220 low hurdles in 22.6 seconds, breaking the world record by 4/10.

When is enough, enough? When the mind says so! In the Olympic games of 1936, he earned four gold medals for:
1) Winning the 100 meter dash.
2) Winning the 200 meter dash.
3) Winning the running broad jump.
4) Being a member of the four man relay team that won that championship race.

When I hear of people who are ready to "throw in the towel", I remember Jesse Owens. He was flesh and blood like you and me, but his ability was empowered by strength of will and love of God. He was examined by doctors who measured his bones, tested his circulation and musculature in order to see if he was Superman, and all they found out was that he was a super man. He died of cancer a number of years ago, but he will always live in my memory as a man to emulate and get inspiration from. I am a better person in every respect from having known him and learned from him.

December 21, 1982

Dear Coach:

A belated happy birthday to you on December 18. The 105 points the team scored against Fairleigh-Dickinson was the frosting on your birthday cake. Talk about totality of offense! We wish you many more birthdays filled with events that make your life meaningful and satisfying. We hope that God grants you your goal this season. As we look at the rest of the season's schedule, it seems that He sent you far more "headaches" than blessings! With God's help, you'll realize the headaches were really blessings in disguise. Recognize a problem as an opportunity. Rise to the occasion, and you'll come out on top. There are many such opportunities for the rest of the '82-83 season—wall to wall!

Remember, body + mind rooted in Spirit = Success! To aid you in keeping goals clearly in view and pursued meaningfully toward accomplishment for holistic/synergistic purposes, please read the following paper, "Making Full Use Of The Power of Holistic Inspiriting". It outlines and explains how to implement a holistic/synergistic program for POSITIVE effect, resulting in devastating consequences—for your opponents! Enjoy and understand this writing as an intended aid for you and the team. Please accept it with our best intentions for the rest of this season as a commitment to you and DePaul.

Read it, Heed it, Proceed with it, and you'll Succeed with it!

While obviously not a substitute for talent, it is the introduction of a divine purpose for drawing out and developing surface and hidden potential, and realizing it in action, thereby effectuating "infectious enthusiasm" that delivers results —*of necessity!*

Back in April, when we met and introduced holism to you, Joey (Coach's son, assistant, and successor) was on a recruiting trip, and we hope that he had a chance to review our thoughts on this subject.

Our purpose, as you know from the outset, is to be of service to you, the team, and the one God who moves us all.

Yours in DePaul,
Norm and Nate

MAKING FULL USE OF THE
POWER OF HOLISTIC INSPIRITING
By
Norm Kozak

'The cure of the part should not be attempted
without treatment of the whole...and
therefore if the head and body are to be
well, you must begin by curing the mind: that
is the first thing.'[1]

When the astronomer Copernicus (1473-1543) proclaimed the sun, rather than the earth, as the center of our solar system, his revolution in astronomy was resisted, challenged, and repeatedly attacked before it was accepted as truth.

Similarly, there is a need for a holistic revolution in consciousness. Instead of mind and body occupying "center stage", with Spirit—the "Divine Energy of Truth and Love" (Sheen, 1953)—being overlaid by them, our task is not to disown the mental and physical, but to have as their basis, Spirit, present in all of their expressions.

When the self is infused with the spirit (Inspiriting) and the striving toward this goal (spirit-mind-body unity) pervades, underlies, and shines through every aspect of holistic total experience, energy-output and efficiency increase—culminating in "peak experiences and performances."

Creating, achieving, and sustaining a holistic mind-set entails five basic steps:

[1] Plato, as quoted in the TM Technigue by Peter Russell (Routledge & Kegan Paul LTD, 1976) p. 77.

1. Knowledge
2. Spiritual act of will
3. Developing a strong, skillful will through will-training and practice.
4. Execution
5. Selective positive reinforcement

KNOWLEDGE

Through the faculty of Intellect, man's understanding of Truth and Love is expanded. He learns that life and love are one, that God's will for him is identical with his real end, and that "all things work together for good to them that love God." With a change in his basic, underlying premises, his motives and behavior change accordingly. These are the inevitable expressions of his outlook on life.

SPIRITUAL ACT OF WILL

Knowledge awakens his Will. The Will answers Yes, No, or Maybe to the possibility of realizing the Divine within himself. The decision he makes must be his own. He is free to go against his Real Spiritual Self, but not free to avoid the consequences if he does so.

DEVELOPING A STRONG, SKILLFUL
WILL THRU WILL TRAINING & PRACTICE

Visualizing to himself and accepting all the past failures, regrets and dilemmas that have resulted from a weak Will or absence of Will, he begins to appreciate the value and possibility of a strong Will capable of preventing their reoccurrence. Imagining all the rewards and opportunities that an efficient Will can produce invigorates the Will to exercise persistence, discipline, and unflagging determination. A skillful Will is one that hits its target, producing the maximum results with the minimum expenditure of energy, in the least amount of time, through "positive imaging". One imagines life-life situations of superior accomplishment. When these occasions become actual, depending on "positive" or "negative" feedback, he either "stays the course" or spontaneously corrects it while "on the march". Moreover, gains consolidated through disciplining the Will militate against backsliding and discouragement.

EXECUTION

According to pragmatism an idea is true if it "works". Its method traces out the consequences of an idea in terms of doing and undergoing. This "courage to risk" is an act of faith, but "faith without works is dead." Perfect love though, being perfect power, "casteth our fear."

SELECTIVE POSITIVE REINFORCEMENT

Unwanted behaviors are dissipated by reinforcement withdrawal, while holistic behaviors are rewarded with emotional payoffs, i.e., sincere approval, praises, compliments, etc.

Beware!!! FALSE PRIDE IS THE ARCH ENEMY OF

HOLISTIC LIVING! In contrast to true, healthy pride based on real accomplishment and established merits, this pride "goeth before a fall," and is No. 1 among the Seven Deadly Sins. It's the "psychic cancer" that must be excised lest it metastasize throughout the entire system. Like Hillel, the great scholar and teacher, we ask, "And if not now, when?"

DePaul University

| Department of Athletics | 1011 West Belden Avenue
Chicago, IL 60614 | 312/321-8010 |

January 27, 1983

Dear Nate:

I have not answered as yet your mail for I have been trying to catch up for months. It seems that all I do is answer mail
all day long. Mail, plus making appearances and public service announcements keep me busy all the time. I am cutting
down on everything to devote more time to coaching.

I won't let anyone or anything take me away from coaching. I really want to help the team. I am trying to make believ-
ers out of the players. It has worked well with.......He believes
he can play. A month ago he couldn't ..... - now he can. He is
confident that he can....I worked with him for a long time to
get him mentally set.

I am working with two other players. At times, I believe I
reached them and then I feel that at times they are out of control......

Well, Nate, we aren't doing as well as we should but we
are in there trying. We are going to beat some good teams
before the season is over.

Yours,

Ray Meyer

February 6, 1983

Dear Coach:

Thanks for taking the time to answer us in this very busy season, especially when the team is on an emotional roller coaster, or, as you recently said, "up and down like a fiddler's elbow." It is noteworthy that you mentioned the word "trying" no less than three times in your letter. We are well assured that you are trying hard to establish the team's attitude. As you well know, trying too hard frequently misses the mark, making matters more difficult. Then trying becomes—"TRYING!" The letter you wrote (October 4, 1982) was written by a man who could anticipate its effects in the face of difficult situations. Reread that letter. You should be proud of your penetrating analysis. Of course, you know we liked it. It is the essence of our lives! Your writing established for us—and we believe in your mind—a causal relationship between state of mind and performance based upon devotion to principle guided by the Almighty, and crowned with satisfying results. Just think of it—we all saw it proven in *Chariots of Fire*!

In the UCLA game you and the team rose to the occasion for the first half. They were beatable and you had them—for one half. That's when we should have utilized the holistic/synergistic approach—applied the October 4 letter!

UCLA has been beaten since with bits and pieces of the holistic knowledge we've shared. Coach, as good as they were, UCLA was shaken by DePaul's ability to control boards and the awesomeness of our potential. Just listen to everyone. It is awesome. But as you note in your latest writing, controlling and using that potential in its proper development has been inconsistent. The kids are performing unreliably. Your writing teaches us that the holistic method had found a home at DePaul. If we need any proof of its applicability to *all*, notice how UCLA, Virginia, and Georgetown are struggling. They certainly have their problems too. Look at what your observations would have done for them. Still, they have a healthy respect for DePaul's potential and it is justified, but not entirely being earned by performance.

The Problem:

How do you convert into positive action the beliefs you expressed October 4, 1982?

The Solution:

You and we have the answer, but the application must be TOTAL, CONSISTENT and not "trying". It is in all the writings, and the UCLA, Illinois State, Pepperdine, Gonzaga, Louisville, St. Joseph's, and Georgetown games.

You and we have the answer and I'm not kidding!

Since a wave cannot be separated from the ocean of which it is a part, and no action exists in isolation from its whole and context, why don't you try to plug in the relational aspect of your team's play to the divine? For as St. Augustine said, "We were born and made for thee, and our hearts are restless till they find peace in thee, O Lord."

A new holistic direction and attitude creates the conditions for consistent peak performances and other significant changes and improvements:

1. Marked reduction in loss of control and anxiety, i.e., "hanging loose" in pressure situations through being problem-solving centered rather than self-centered.
2. More accurate perception and greater clarity in thought.
3. True pride and joy in accomplishment and achievement.

Coach, God bless you and here's hoping your New Year's wish—an NCAA Tournament invitation—comes true. It is still within your grasp but you and the team must take it! Let's sit down early one morning now and see how to TAKE IT! It's not hard and everyone is wondering why we are having such a hard time; let's show them how easy it is! It is essentially in the October 4 letter!

Warm regards,
Norm Kozak
Nathan Yellen

February 21, 1983

Dear Coach:

I asked Pat (Coach's secretary) to give you my message— to read once again our last letter to you. Sunday's loss (St. John's) proved the applicability of my message. We've got it —everyone knows we've got it; every team FEARS our ability and is surprised that we fail in its practical application.

You have five days before Notre Dame to bring LIFE to this team and it is more than enough time. Nothing difficult, certainly understandable and so easy to do. It's all in our last letter and your letter of October 4, 1982.

*Do well against the Irish! Have breakfast with us, Coach, it will help! I promise you that.

> Warm regards,
> Nate

---

*DePaul defeated Notre Dame 55-53 on an 18-foot beat-the-buzzer basket by Kenny Patterson.

The 1982-83 Basketball Season was not, sadly for the holistic approach, a glorious application of its principles at DePaul University. Even though Coach Ray agreed our program was sound, measurable results did not occur...problems, personalities, compulsion, fears—whatever!

Talking and writing about what needs to be done is one thing; doing it is another. We wanted "working holism" to complement theoretical discussion immediately, on a consistent basis and with conclusive results (probably more than we could or should have realistically expected). But, short of "planned execution", we were confident that a holistic model provided by Coach himself (after all, God was not an afterthought to Coach but the core of his life) could influence the kids to use God's power—the sleeping giant within—indirectly, if not directly, to achieve VICTORY. Earlier Ray wrote that he was thinking of ways to join basketball and holism, and we believed him. But even if one knows the "what for?", the goal, one doesn't always know the "how to", the way to the goal. Coach would have to decide for himself how to put holism to work in his particular situation; but if he wanted our help we were there.

The season's end was near. The next (42nd) would be Ray's last. This was weighing on his mind, in addition to his life after coaching. To get a sixth straight NCAA Tournament bid and bring his weight under control were of immediate importance.

Coach still felt his Demons had a chance, however slight, to go to the NCAA tourney if they could win convincingly over the Dayton Flyers, a team they had beaten earlier at the Rosemont Horizon. But the dream was short-lived. DePaul didn't play well and lost 80-71.

Nevertheless, the team did receive and accept a National Invitational Tournament (NIT) bid for post-season play.

In the opening round they (the Demons) bested a dogged Minnesota team 76-73 (the lead seesawed back and forth no less than five times in the final minute); then on a last second (buzzer) 35-foot shot by Kenny Patterson they slipped past the Wildcats of Northwestern, 65-63. Against Mississippi they literally stole (16 steals) the game, winning 75-67.

The holistic doctrine took on a special meaning with the saying "break your opponent early; take them out of the game and then enjoy the game"—a sure sign of VICTORY.

March 26, 1983

Dear Coach:

This will be our last communication with you until you come home from New York (Madison Square Garden) with the team, and the FINAL FOUR, TWO, AND ONE! All the way—one game at a time. This is what you are there to *do* and that alone. Not for school, boys, you, or love of game, but because you and the boys must use your God-given talents to the best of your ability to achieve. This tournament is yours and yours alone to take, but you must take it!

Play "AS IF" you are No. 1 and you will become No. 1! God love you, care for you and the team. With that, what else does one need? BREAK THEM (Nebraska) EARLY, SIGNIFI-CANTLY, and FINALLY. THEN ENJOY THE GAME!

> Warmest regards,
> Norm and Nate

Tyrone Corbin saved DePaul in their semifinal win over Nebraska. He garnered 16 rebounds and had 15 points in the Demons 65-58 victory. But in the championship game DePaul shot poorly (25 of 74) and was defeated by Fresno State 69-60.

April 22, 1983

Dear Coach:

I will be at Chicamouga battlefield or fishing in the Ozarks when you get this letter, but I had to mark the passage of one year since you met Norm and I. How much we've learned from you to aid us in our interest in holism/synergism, and the understanding and respect of you that we acquired from your candid and forthright discussions with us. Thanks for all you've done, including this week's meeting when you signed our prints with a kind personal note.

DO something about your weight NOW, and get on a program NOW! If you can't do it yourself positively, call........at ....He will "insult" you appropriately, as he did me to get in gear and LOSE (weight, that is!). Be well and warm regards to your family.

God Love You,
Nate

DePaul University

Department of Athletics   1011 West Belden Avenue   312/321-8010
                                 Chicago, IL 60614

May 24, 1983

Dear Nate:

I want to thank you for your nice letter and your kind thoughts. I do appreciate your friendship.

My health is fine. I have to sit around and do nothing for another week and then I will be off and running. I don't like sitting around the house and doing nothing. This is the most difficult part of the operation (medical). It is so boring. Thank God for television and all the sports on it. It really does help to pass the time away...

Ray Meyer

October 11, 1983

Dear Coach:

It's another October and another basketball season. We wish you a successful one in which all that is sought by you is achieved. It is going to be a most memorable season filled with milestones, and hopefully without millstones! It is awesome to contemplate 700 victories and the capping of a lifetime devoted selflessly to this game and excellence in this, your last season as active coach. The words fairly choke in our mouths—last season of Ray Meyer. But the seeming finality of active coaching is not at all finality. In this season you have the rarest of opportunities to leave a legacy of YOU that can shine with all your past successes and problems, and place all in a proper perspective.

The truly testing schedule with a ten-man squad is the stuff of which legends are made. Rising to occasion in response to your last season can create a deep feeling of satisfaction, motivation and reward, that can launch Joey and the team into the "post-Coach" era. So much to be gained, done, and achieved. It all faces you. You are properly equipped to "pull it off". You will be tested as never before. In many cases your response will of necessity be new—yes—new, but according to principle! Your faith, spirit, knowledge, and drive are all that are needed to do it. God knows we would be willing to assist you in any way you wish. We are your friends!

Recalling your love of baseball we close in mentioning the peak performance season of pitcher John Denny (19 wins, 6 losses), probable Cy Young Award winner of the Philadelphia Phillies who, for some reason obscure to most of the blind world rose from 0-2 with the Phillies last season. There is always a reason and you as usual know—the state of mind influenced by his becoming a born-again Christian. The old equation: God + mind + body = success. How many times have you and we said "that is all that counts"? It must be this holistic/synergistic approach that was the basis of his new attitude that put him, literally, over the top; removing him from the obscurity of nonperformance to "the bright light of day", while performance with purpose was his goal and reward. This challenge faces all of us and for all our goodness, the choice must still be positively made. "Choose Life," saith the Lord—adversity and all; for that is what produces things that last and are worthwhile. We can't help but think that you are in a most unique, creative situation to give the world a lesson in how a man, already honored, rose yet one more time against adversity to prove this synergistic principle.

Warmest regards to the team, Joey, all the coaches, DePaul, Marge, and you; last, but far from least! May the Almighty grant all that you see before you.

God Love You,
Nate & Norm

October 16, 1983

Dear Coach:

Two days ago, the Chicago Sun-Times wrote about the University of Illinois football players turning to "Imagery" inside a dark room, a pre-game strategy designed to bring the ability-level of the mind to the same level as the body. Is this what it's all about? The Illinois players think they have defined the problem, but is "dark room imagery" a real, permanent solution? The team's record shows that its permanency is, as yet, unproven.

"What we try to do," says Dan Smith, Illinois sports psychologist, "is raise those psychological levels to match the physical levels." However, what is really needed is to raise the psychological level to the spiritual level. Then the body reaches and performs at that level, too.

The Chicago White Sox turned to hypnotism and Fran Tarkenton's "School for Winning". They won their division, but UGLY. In the playoffs, they failed with a seemingly indestructible hitting attack. The Sox are looking forward to another Western Division Championship in 1984, but in reality, they have the fight of their lives on their hands, with no assurance of victory. These two very recent events caused me to think back, and upon reflection with Norm, I had to write you today.

A year and one-half ago, after the Athletes In Action game, we met with you regarding a Holistic Basketball program.

Your October 1982 letter ranks you as one of its adherents, but its consistent use for positive results must be yet unclear in your mind. *Chariots of Fire* was living proof of its validity; now UCLA is commencing a mental conditioning program.

Norm and I would like to bring such a program into being; we feel it would be demoralizing to any opponent. It had been and is our hope that you would allow us to help you with such a plan, because we do believe that you accept its reality, applicability, and chance for success. God knows, DePaul faces an awesome schedule this "Last Hurrah" active season of yours, and such a program would be a positive aid to the team. You not only believe in the tenets and goals of our program, but you know what is on our minds and in our hearts: the use of the power and talent within each of us to run a straight race, to the best of our ability, for the gratification of God! Unbeatable, permanent, uplifting, inspiring, and DOABLE!

Dear friend—let's have breakfast or meet one more time if your concur with our evaluation. It's really not difficult to do and make it work, if you believe. What are you positively doing to bring into fruition the conditions that you so articulately enumerate in that October 1982 letter? Let's at least look at it so you can hear what we have in mind.

God Love You,
Nathan Yellen

P.S. Note what the Chicago Tribune (October 9, 1983) wrote: Larussa" (Tony, White Sox manager) "mentioned that they" —(Orioles) "do the little things so well that it becomes really a big thing. Others have said that Baltimore's whole is what shoots you dead, not the sum of its parts." Sound familiar, Coach?

DePaul University

Department of Athletics   1011 West Belden Avenue   312/321-8010
                                 Chicago, IL 60614

October 24, 1983

Dear Nathan:

I enjoyed reading the material you sent me lately. I am getting a lot of material on positive mental conditioning. There are a number of people here in Chicago who want to work with our players. They have classes in mental conditioning...we have to be careful.

You and Norm are truly interested in helping our athletes. I have been taking a lot of advice from you and your articles. It is beginning to rub off on our athletes.

I will try to arrange a breakfast with you and Norm. Maybe in a couple of weeks we will get together. I have a new book, *The Winning Edge*, and it contains quotes of some of our famous athletes. They all prepared themselves mentally and positively.

Nate, the season will be a good one. We are beginning to progress. We have an intra-squad scrimmage and then we play the European team. After that we will know where we are.

Yours,

Ray Meyer

October 27, 1983

Coach Ray Meyer
DePaul University
Chicago, Illinois 60614

Dear Coach:

Few communications received by me in this life have made me happier or filled me with a greater sense of satisfaction than the one I got from you on October 24, 1983. Most notably, upon reading it and absorbing its contents, my reaction was that here, about a year and a half after you, Norm and I spoke about the principles, benefits, and methods of holistic/synergistic living, you are facing with confidence the prospect of the institution of some program that seeks the integration of spirit, mind, and body for the purpose of bringing more meaning to the performance of athletes. I call that progress! You yourself have made great strides in this area that brings the ultimate gratification and reward: self-control for purpose! If not so—what do you ascribe your loss of 20+ pounds to? Are you planning to enter the Mr. America contest for a beautiful body? I think not. Your desire for total well-being is very much in evidence to us. This is what is facing you now.

Your October 1982 letter, although none of us knew it then, laid down the criteria by which any mind-control plan that you employed would be judged, and while Norm and I were pleased then that you agreed with us in principle, and we agreed with that letter, there was no impetus for its installation. Now, all of us know why it is required and its importance—NOW! Getting back to this week's letter, you used the term "positive mental conditioning" that a few people who wish to work with your players are selling in Chicago. They employ hypnotism, "dark rooms", "School of Winning", and various techniques that seek to alter the mental process and thereby change behavior. Their intentions are good and these techniques frequently produce immediate results. But how many of them stand the test of time? What causes a smoker to finally quit; a drinker to stop drinking finally, and an eater to finally moderate his eating? Self-determined, goal-oriented implemented mental conditioning based on real purposes is always the only answer that can be permanent—all else is temporary and crisis generally tests these systems to the limit. You know how to judge these people who wish to institute "positive mental conditioning"; your October 1982 letter tells you! Look at the Sox debacle and the turnabout of pitcher John Denny, and we know that you know! "Positive mental conditioning" is but one aspect of the problem; but it doesn't go far enough. *Chariots of Fire* showed the right principles in action; it gave us a true story to illustrate them, and we all spoke of this a year and one-half ago!

The sole reason that you took our advice in the intervening time is that it appealed to you and was in accord with

God's plan, explaining further why you felt good about it and spoke with us again and again. It, most assuredly, also explains why we sought further to be of assistance to you. We believed you were not an "our team plays" type of coach, but rather an "our team plays and wins!" type, looking for a method to enforce this plan. You know what a working program must encompass and how to judge what anyone seeks to implement as to workability and applicability. Knee-jerk reaction is not thinking; "WINNING UGLY" is not VICTORY; false pride is not the pride God wishes for us. Victorious, synergistic living is EVERYTHING! You can see it in Denny, Willie Stargell, Ernie Banks, Terry Cummings, ad infinitum. But unless spiritual force becomes self-sustaining, it needs to be continually recalled and revived, or else the mind slips back to what it was.

On that day in April, 1982, we spoke of universals—not just helpful actions; we spoke of self-induced control (with God's guidance) aided by measurement of progress. We had with you that day, a glimpse into eternity; if not, why are we still talking to one another?

We must be together again; now—any hour of day or night, any place, any question, any topic—no holds barred. You must know how to articulate what you want and judge what is placed before you, and we must show you what we can do for you with predictable results. You already know what is in our minds and in our hearts. We can aid you immeasurably in surveying this field so you can separate weed from wheat, temporary good from permanent, and form from substance.

Your observance that the practices must be coordinated, worthwhile, and progressive has been the hallmark of Norm's life and mine for over 33 years. But if the practices are not right in the beginning, the games won't be right in the end. We wish CONCLUSIVENESS for the goals that we have shared in our writings and conversations, and I must invite your positive call. It has been our pleasure to be of assistance to you during this time in whatever way you found us so. Now you must know what we want for you, the team, and DePaul. It is a worthy project. Please contact us before you do anything final.

> God Love You,
> Nathan Yellen

October 29, 1983

Coach Ray Meyer
DePaul University
1011 West Belden Avenue
Chicago, Illinois 60614

Dear Coach:

As you put it, it's absolutely true that Nathan and I are interested in helping your athletes, but in writing this letter to you I'm trying to be self-transcending because I believe unselfish love "seeketh not its own."

I'm gratified that our advice is starting to rub off on your athletes. Coach, regarding the material you've been getting on positive mental conditioning, my personal advice to you is to avoid any program unless it includes the vertical dimension —the dimension that pointeth upward to God.

Though B.F. Skinner, the founder of "Operant Conditioning", the offspring of reinforcement theory, taught *pigeons* how to play Ping-Pong through the establishment of a positive reward system, "*Man* does not live by bread alone" and needs, as William James said, "Something More."

It's not that the positive conditioning programs don't have some merits; they certainly do. But these are only window dressing and a Band-Aid approach for they deal with the horizontal dimension of living only, and unless they are included within a holistic context and framework, the benefits from these conditioning programs won't be lasting.

Advising the Ephesians, Saint Paul once said, "Having done all, stand." You will—with a holistic solution to your complex problem.

God Bless You,
Your friend,
Norm Kozak

November 2, 1983

Coach Ray Meyer
DePaul University
1011 West Belden Avenue
Chicago, Illinois 60614

Dear Coach:

When the schedule came out for DePaul's 1983-84 Basketball Season, a quick examination disclosed that over 40 percent of the teams we play could be among the "top 20". Another 30 percent are "trouble-giving" good teams that make the game more than just interesting. Most of the balance will be a good game. We do not run from "class opponents". That is clear. Norm and I looked at this schedule months ago and thought little of it until last night when we decided to go to the intra-squad game. Who knows, with all the illness and injuries, if it will be a game? It was then that memories of the Athletes In Action game started to flood my mind. I came to the following conclusion.

I finally drew the conclusion that the Czech National Team (next on our schedule) is the ANTITHESIS of the Athletes In Action squad. Where "Athletes" were most notably SYNERGIC (devoted body, mind, and spirit to God), the Czech team is ATHEISTIC—Godless, if you will! For the Czechs, spirit is not a religious concept, but a dimension of meaning and purpose that excludes God and debases Him! They are, by design and choice, cut off from the ULTIMATE LIFE-GIVING source of all goodness and cause for meaningful existence. They can, by seeking professional excellence and motivating themselves, become HOLISTIC—but they cannot, by definition, be SYNERGISTIC as was Eric Liddell in *Chariots of Fire*. In this observation I found great meaning related to the 1982 "Athletes" game. In that game we played a team that *"prayed* and *played"*—who can ever forget the impact of them on that crowd and the team? The opening and mid-game praying and feeling that "God was on their side" enforced the concept that they could knock off the NUMBER ONE TEAM IN AMERICA—and they did! They did it using SYNERGIC principles without doubt and what is more, they beat us: A CATHOLIC SCHOOL, devoted mind, body, and spirit to GOD! This was a portent of things to come and you are living them now.

In a short time we will be up against the Czech team of "professionals", presumably playing as hard as they can against a "God-saturated Catholic Institution" that you and I are proud and devoted to; but what strength to be drawn from God will be exhibited against the Godless to aid our athletes in the competition? Will we be synergic against the Godless, or will we face them non-synergic, as we faced Athletes In Action synergy? As I see it, we have in this game all that Norm and I have tried to convey to you in this past one and one-half years—that synergy is what we must practice, breathe, and LIVE if we wish to compete and WIN WITH PURPOSE! With 11 men, injuries, illness, and the problems of the season, God is our most valuable ally, as He is, was, and always will be! Recalling the Athletes In Action game, we cannot afford to throw away any advantages against any Godless team.

Moses faced the power and wrath of Pharaoh and Godless Egypt with only a staff and the power of God behind and surrounding him. His story serves as a timeless example of "he who completely and selflessly serves the Lord shall be protected and exalted above his opponents." By God, Moses had his day! He trusted in God when he took on Numero Uno just as we did in our Revolution from England and prevailed, through the difficult times, trusting in God and working, performing, and DOING. Is this the spirit and determination that we will employ this season against the Czech team or will we just love God and draw nothing from the special relationship that He shares with mankind? Remember, Athletes In Action did this to us!

I hope as always, that this is helpful to you, but there are too many things to say in writing that we wish further to convey to you. We await your call to a meeting—ANYTIME, ANYPLACE.

God Love You,
Nathan Yellen

November 4, 1983

Dear Coach:

The depiction of "The Tree of Life" in this card says so much of what I feel about life. It is a course of strength to those who hold fast to it! God teaches us that, but WE must CHOOSE LIFE! The negative naysayers look for ill. We must look for and find good. It's hard, but we must find it in adversity and distractions. Your weight loss told me that you are taking control of yourself. The consideration of the introduction of a positive motivation system tells me more. Continue and God love you for it!

Paul Valery, the essayist, said, "The trouble with our times is that the future is not what it used to be." The future will be what we make it today, positively for good; if negatively, we will get what is undone, ignored, or pursued for a useless purpose.

God Love You,
Nate

PLAY BALL

As the 1983-84 Basketball Season, the Coach's last, was about to get under way, demands on his time increased from all directions. In the face of everything pulling at him at once, the control that he attained at the close of last season needed to continue. His weight was still dropping and he felt well, but would he pick up and DO what we eagerly wanted for him and the team?

The exhibition game with the Godless, holistic Czech team, in which we hoped synergy would be used to defeat holism—God over the godless—was an acid test, as we saw it. Guess what? DePaul lost in overtime, and the team was not defeated; it lost! In the Athletes In Action game, DePaul was synergically beaten by a God-driven team, and now against the Czechs was beaten holistically by a Godless team. A God-centered university should not suffer such losses—yet it did! Was this a portent of games to follow? We knew that a TEAM was in the making and had faith in the Coach.

DePaul University

Department of Athletics   1011 West Belden Avenue   312/321-8010
                                 Chicago, IL 60614

November 15, 1983

Dear Norm,

Thanks for your letter and the "Tree of Life" (card). You and Nate are very good friends. There is nothing I do that I have not looked upward to God. He is the focal point of all of my activities.

In little ways here and there, I am getting the idea across to the players. They are developing a very healthy attitude toward athletics and life itself. It is going to be a very long year for me. There are so many people coming around with substantial financial offers to have me do things for them.

I want to coach this year and I want to do the best job I can. There are so many distractions that I would like to avoid. My whole thoughts will be devoted to my job. This is all I am concerned with. I have to practice now.

Yours,
Ray Meyer

November 22, 1983

Dear Ray:

With everything you have to do, we certainly and most deeply appreciate your last note. It seems to us in reading between the lines, that in your mind the "offers" and so-called "do-gooders for Ray Meyer" are deflecting your attention from your coaching of the DePaul Blue Demons for the entire 1983-84 season. We believe you are producing the best team possible and working with the athletes to develop them. But because of what you have been exposed to, namely the offers, you feel that there is a divided loyalty and you really wish the "Ray Meyer" part of this season would go away. But it will not, we are happy to say! You must put out of your mind the notion that the "Ray Meyer" part must be squelched or stopped in order for you to do your work. This is not true. Read on.

In April 1984 the "Ray Meyer on his own" part of your life will begin. After the NCAA Tournament and 42 years of coaching 700+ victories under your belt, you, Ray, storyteller, teacher, lover of basketball and life will begin a new life in control of what you have made of yourself—a walking, talking, real Hall of Fame legend and valuable property! This situation must be faced and resolved, not shunted aside. It is plain for us, standing next to you, to see. You must disenthrall

yourself from handling this matter and stop punishing yourself by believing you are not doing your job. Concentrate
instead on the good that you have done for so many kids and
for God's sake.

In order for the "Ray Meyer on his own" part of your life
to get rolling, lead time is needed by the "offer givers" and
understandably that time is now. Their motives are many and
varied, but they need time to prepare for endorsements,
appearances, etc., and you need time for "your people" to
consider what is "right" for you—that time is now also. Get
yourself competent advisers to sift through the "offers" and,
based upon their knowledge of you and your wishes, have
them select and recommend in final form what is worthy of
your approval. Pure and simple! What we are telling you is
real, DOABLE, and there are people around who are extreme-
ly qualified and have interest in you in friendship.

Another point: Your life in 1984 independent of DePaul is
necessary for Joey to establish himself. This does not mean
that your 42 year affiliation with DePaul is ended; not at all.
You and DePaul will be physically separated, and attached
spiritually and emotionally, but not economically; that is
nothing to fear. It is an opportunity to get closer to, yet independent of, DePaul. Strong, healthy, and separate!

Remember Mark (Aguirre) and Terry (Cummings), (former DePaul All-Americans), began their "life after DePaul"
while they were still there; but you can manage this transition
better and we will help you, if you wish. What is important is

that you separate "Ray Meyer, valuable property" from "Ray Meyer, coach", and by the appropriate methods "manage" both; doing both well. You take the coaching and get "managers" who manage to take care of "Ray Meyer" so he can, in addition to doing his job, make meaningful decisions affecting his life after and away from DePaul, but in spirit, ever there!

We hope this makes sense to you because we believe in it, and it comes from the best source we know of: mind, love, and friendship born of a 19-month-old meeting where we found that you and we share a number of common interests. Remarkable indeed! Friendship grew from all of it, and it extends to Joey too!

> God Love You,
> Norm Kozak
> Nathan Yellen

P.S. Happy Thanksgiving to you and yours and may The Good Lord fill your cup to the brim with love, health, and friendship!

DePaul University

Department of Athletics   1011 West Belden Avenue   312/321-8010
Chicago, IL 60614

November 30, 1983

Dear Nate:

I am really trying to put everything out of my mind but coaching. I find it very hard to do business with all the daily bustle and distractions around here. Yes, I have turned over all outside activities....I want to coach—I would like to please everyone but that is impossible. I know my first duty and love is coaching. I am going to worry about my life after coaching when that time comes.

As soon as I am through with all the activities around here, I am going away for a couple of weeks. When I return, then I will worry about the next step in my life.

Thanks for your letter!

Ray

A year and a half later, but then it happened: the first holistic game! Too much had transpired between Coach and Us for the holistic attitude not to take hold and issue in action. Not only was Ohio University "taken out" of the game and "kept out", but the team was "blown out". Unmistakable CONTROL, FIRE AND TOTALITY of TEAM that we were looking for! Danny Nee, the Ohio coach, likened himself to General George Custer during his "last stand" at Little Big Horn; only it wasn't Indians coming at Coach Nee and his team, but Demons!

This was some birthday: The birth of HOLISTIC BAS-KETBALL, and Ray was the Father; yet this holistic "resource" was barely being tapped, and certainly not via any organized, planful procedure. Our question was this: If the message transmitted without the use of words was so power-ful, how awesome would it have been if the philosophy of holism was directly communicated and INTERNALIZED through open, free-flowing dialogue, so that it was CON-SCIOUSLY lived? Just the thought of it boggled our minds.

What concerned Us was whether the holistic "game plan" would be consistently reinforced and acquire motor power. Otherwise, we feared the gains wouldn't be permanent and the Demons could slip back. We were also worried that they might become too prideful and set themselves up for a "fall". Could they go all the way or even reach the Final Four in the NCAA tourney with holism inside their heads, but lacking depth, because it was outside their awareness and understanding? We hoped so; they certainly had the talent. But the Bible tells us: "The race is not to the swift, nor the battle to the strong" (Eccles. 9:11). We saw the need for the underlying, holistic foundation to become more forceful.

It was with this thought in mind that Nate wrote Coach the following amusing story. Its message was intended to raise Coach's awareness of the *importance* and *necessity* of using "working holism" so that the team wouldn't suffer a downfall.

WHAT ARE WE WAITING FOR?

There was a preacher whose faith in God was so strong that at any crossroad or problem in his life, he would kneel down and pray to God for help, and wait till He would show him the way out of his difficult situation. The preacher believed that God would always send an answer, and he preached this message to all his parishioners regularly. The message was his life's purpose.

There came to his town a devastating rainfall, and after nine consecutive days of it, there was great concern for the total flooding and ruin of the community, as there seemed to be no relief in sight. He urged his parishioners not to let up in their prayers and to ask God for guidance in deciding whether to remain or leave. The water level rose steadily and after the first floor of his home was under water, a boat sailed by with friends urging him to flee. He said, "God will send me a reply and deliverance from this catastrophe," so they sailed off leaving him on the second landing of his house with the rain still falling.

Two days later, a second boat with friends and parishioners came to him while he was perched precariously on his tiptoes, stumbling on the roof of his house, and he told them that he would remain, as ever, waiting for God's response. Later that morning, still others in a helicopter found him in the downpour on his chimney, and implored him to come with them. "No," he said, "I'll wait for the good Lord's instruction!" And they flew away sadly.

The preacher drowned and upon arriving in Heaven and finding it even more beautiful than he had ever imagined, he asked to speak with God, and was granted that request. "Good Lord," he said, "why did You forsake me and leave me with no program or plan to save me from the rain, when You knew I loved You and trusted in You so completely? Didn't I always ask for Your guidance in all I was troubled over? Why did You send me no answer?"

The Lord replied, "You darn fool, I sent you two boats and a helicopter, didn't I?"

December 1, 1983

Dear Coach Ray:

I got your note and was pleased to learn that all of your personal post-season life has been delegated to competent hands. It sounds as if they are experienced. You should get much better results using these folks. They will look out for your interests. Most important.

Talk about controlling destiny and creating good, teamy feelings—this game was one in a million! By God, you must be floating after the way the kids played against Ohio! DePaul intimidated and controlled a taller team. Your players performed under control and played with precision and meaning. Now they must play this way 32 more times this season.

Kenny P. (Patterson) was faster than quick and he was simply holism incarnate. You must keep him under control all the time, and he will become the pro that he has within him. Holmes (Kevin), Comegys (Dallas), Corbin (Tyrone), McMillan (Jerry), Jackson (Tony), and Lampley (Lemone)—God love him—were dynamite.

It was an exhilarating and exciting game, but it was even more. It was a holistic success because the TEAM effort was greater than the sum of the individual performances, and you could see, feel, and know it! The team was on fire holistically!

You are to be congratulated. This is what it's all about. Keep it up. Now for Illinois State! Break them early and keep them broken!

God Love You All,
Norm and Nate

The Ohio University game was DePaul's second victory of the regular season. In the opener, the Demons won over Northern Illinois by 15 points. Although Victory No. 700 over Illinois State on December 2, 1983, at the Rosemont Horizon gave Coach great personal satisfaction, he called it his "second-biggest thrill." Coach now became a Member of the 700 Club. Only four others before him reached this milestone: Adolph Rupp (Kentucky), Phog Allen (Kansas), Henry "Hank" Iba (Oklahoma State), and Ed Diddle of Western Kentucky.

Coach's biggest thrill was getting to the Final Four of the NCAA Tournament by defeating UCLA in 1979. The 1978-79 season was also marked by his induction into the National Basketball Hall of Fame. The following season (1979-80), however, the Bruins of UCLA redeemed themselves by knocking off DePaul in the NCAA tourney.

Soon afterward, on April 24, 1980, Mark Aguirre, the team's number one player, resolved his dilemma of whether to turn professional or stay in school. You may be surprised to learn that the motivating force behind Mark's decision to remain at DePaul was Love. Mark said that more than money and the pro league he loved Coach and his teammates. He realized that the love he was getting at DePaul was nowhere else to be found. Amen on that.

December 8, 1983

Dear Coach Ray:

This was a most illuminating and conclusive period of one week's time! The Ohio game was the first holistic game we ever witnessed; one of DePaul's best of all time—and everyone knows it! The team play and totality of effort was larger than the sum of the individual performances, which were terrific. Victories No. 700 and No. 701 are behind you with the 24 point spread over Western Michigan. Your personal economics are handled by people whose competence you trust in; nice to see your life is under control and you are back to coaching —great!

Now, Georgetown is in front of you. They can be had—a la Ohio. This game is up your alley and you know how to do it. We're excited for you and wish you the best. This is your season of control and coaching!

God Love You and the Kids,
Norm and Nate

A leading sportscaster said on national TV that an athlete has to have a certain amount of "inner arrogance" to be successful. To us, inner arrogance characterizes the state of mind or attitude of an athlete who is *supremely* confident, yet not overconfident. Such an athlete takes charge in "clutch" situations and does not fear failure. He expects to win but does not take winning for granted.

In our opinion, in the game between DePaul and Georgetown, Georgetown took DePaul for granted. Their players were confident—but to a fault! The year before, DePaul lost by six points to the Hoyas of Georgetown at Georgetown. But in Saturday night's game, DePaul, after trailing by 15 points, narrowed the gap to ten as the first half ended. The Demons "stayed hungry", never gave up, and at the end of regulation time the third-ranked Hoyas were upset 63-61. The Hoyas humbled themselves by the "backslide of false pride".

DePaul was scheduled to play next in Japan. The flight was sure to be joyous.

December 11, 1983

Dear Ray:

Good to have Georgetown out of the way. Just a few thoughts for Japan that are on our minds regarding this most unique season.

It started with the loss to Godless Czechoslovakia that used HOLISM to beat us—we dominated them though they were taller, and we lost though we are a Christian university. What an anomaly—an enigma from which you and the team came back to play the first HOLISTIC game in DePaul history against Ohio. In our minds, that game will live forever as a VICTORY, not just a win.

Now you are going to Japan whose culture does not embrace the Judeo-Christian concept of ONE GOD, but bases holism upon ancestral values and the Shinto-Buddhist religions. These two thoughts awaken in us the great source of our strength, to be tapped in order to project our WILL for positive purposes. You and we believe, trust, and MOVE under the Judeo-Christian concept, and that gives us the indomitable faith needed to succeed; but for God's purposes. Hold to this Tree of Life and continue to make it work for you and all! *Chariots of Fire* is real and it LIVES!

Do well in Japan, knowing that our minds and hearts, as ever, are with you. Please read the *Power For Living* book (a paperback about famous athletes and people who regard God, not themselves, as No. 1) and see if you feel it might be helpful to_____. God love that kid. EVERYONE is with him and wants him to do what he clearly is capable of Doing! What do you think of the book, Coach? It may be of great use to you.

Take care and God Love You,
Norm and Nate

December 14, 1983

Dear Friend and Coach:

Congratulations on your victory over Georgetown and may your 70th birthday be your healthiest and happiest ever.

I know you're having a lot of "peak experiences", and my aim in this letter is to enable you to experience more of them. God knows, as you so aptly put it, you've been "up and down like a fiddler's elbow."

The Hoyas of Georgetown sealed their fate at the start of the second half. They came out and played all "puffed up". They had the "pride that goeth before a fall," and the "haughtiness that ends in disaster and compulsion"—the enemy of the holistic attitude and approach.

Your team had the true pride and intensity that ends in joy and accomplishment—the Holistic, Synergistic State of Mind. Since "eternal vigilance is the price of freedom," my suggestion to you, Coach, and the decision always rests with yourself, is to be constantly watchful of the aforementioned "inner enemy": false pride. This is a no-no—a red flag! Don't allow this third opponent—the other two being the team you're playing and the clock—to become a part of your team's play.

Another thing, Coach, when you speak of intensity, you may be putting the "cart before the horse". Cognitive therapist Harold D. Werner (1982) said that the intensity of a person's behavior depends on how strong his will is. May (1969), defined will as "the capacity to organize one-self...toward a certain goal..." Arousing, strengthening, training, and developing the will to "want it (VICTORY) badly enough," powered by self-generated motivation, is the key to "intensity of behavior."

Good luck in Japan; try to impress upon the players not to slacken their efforts when they're ahead, but at that time to lower the boom and deliver the K.O. punch.

Warmest regards,
Norm Kozak

December 18, 1983

Dear Ray:

Happy Birthday (number 70) to you. Congratulations on winning in the Suntory Ball in Japan. It's good to have Japan out of the way and the second 7 — 700 victories, 70 years of age. There's a kicker in Purdue; a few wrinkles and a BURN-ING DESIRE with ability to stop us. Enough said. It's good to have you back and especially in the Christmas Season. Do well with Purdue—nothing less than the holistic triumph of Ohio and G-Town, but strive for synergy. Accept no less and you'll get no less.

Your direction of the kids' efforts to please the Almighty could be infectious. Showing *Chariots of Fire* again could affect the kids remarkably and give new meaning now.

Along with the backing of the crowd, the "sixth man" to spark the team, you can have the Spirit of God hovering over the game floor. Playing the music from *Chariots of Fire* in the locker room before the game, during warm-ups, and at the start of the second half reminds the kids of their task and desire to accomplish as a team for God! Positive results would follow. The power of synergy can make this season, the culmination of 42 years, live forever as dedicated to God!

We would like to have breakfast with you for one hour on

Monday morning, December 26, (no work). We have some things that you must see and hear in order to appreciate. Call_____ or _____.

God Love You,
Nathan Yellen

A TRUE STORY

Ray, only you know how much Norm and I are devoted to holistic/synergic life and principles. Last week we were considering Mark Aguirre (Dallas Mavericks) and the fabulous statistics that he is amassing now. He is unstoppable and impossible to deal with. The numbers in recent weeks are beyond belief and he is not done yet! It is no secret that we considered him neither holistic nor synergic. Terry (Cummings) is synergic and many are holistic. But Mark in all his time at DePaul and in the NBA (National Basketball Association) was just a great, natural talent.

This year, however, his play is better than ever and different in quality—HE IS ON FIRE! Why? In addition to having a great teacher and coach, Dick Motta, we learned from a friend that Mark was "born again"! So what else is new? The fire that he has now is God's fire from *Chariots of Fire*, and if 24 points per game and extraordinary rebounding were sufficient before—look at what he is doing now!!! CONSISTENTLY UNDER CONTROL WHILE TAKING HIS TEAM TO THE TOP! I'll bet that he is one happy human being now, and could be helpful to_____, who appears like a lost, sensitive, and bright young man who should be able to make peace with himself and become the best he can be. You have the book (*Power For Living*) with its examples and method. If_____ finds his way, his enthusiasm could infect the entire team and

only God knows where it would all end—games like Ohio
and Georgetown could be the rule rather than the exception.

PRACTICE, PRACTICE, PRACTICE

Even though DePaul was 7-0 and ranked fourth nationally, Coach wasn't happy with his Demons' performance in Japan, and planned a practice following the team's arrival in Chicago.

What about practice? Does practice make perfect? We're learning a lot from Walter Downing, a former DePaul player, who transferred to Marquette University to play his last two years. Walter said, "...Well, practice does not make perfect. It just makes more permanent our imperfections." Good observation, Walter. It makes us wonder how often teams are practicing "things right", but not practicing the "right things". It was in this vein, seven months later, that Coach Ray, at the Illinois State Bar Association Annual Meeting, added:

It's not the length of practice, but the quality of practice...Talent is not enough...You can measure talent, but you can't measure heart.

By "heart" is intended human "WILL" in this instructive saying from Proverbs 3:1 in the Bible: "My son, forget not my teaching. But let thy *heart* keep my commandment" (italics added).

Developing a strong, skillful and good will in PRACTICE cannot be too strongly emphasized. You see it in Larry Bird, now starring for the Boston Celtics. He's WILLING to go to any length to keep himself and his team "on top". He puts "umph" into his WILL by engaging in a "one-man shoot-around" an hour ahead of the game. At game time his Will is all fired up. Since perfection is not humanly possible, practice does not make perfect—but it makes us more perfect if we practice the "right things", with the right attitude, in the right way, and for the right reasons.

December 21, 1983

Dear Coach:

It seems as if Purdue possibly forgot about Evansville (and lost) on its way to play DePaul, tomorrow. It still holds true—one game at a time! We still have a couple of months to worry about Evansville, but let's give Purdue the Ohio/Georgetown program: total attack and defense. Purdue is no "schlep" and they're waiting for us.

We hope that you've recovered from "jet lag" (Japan). I found myself irritable coming home from Europe. I hope all is well with the kids. Break Purdue as early as you can—and keep them broken! TEAMINESS will do it. Have a good holiday!

God Love You and the TEAM!
Norm and Nate

Tyrone Corbin scored a career-high 24 points in DePaul's 68-61 victory over Purdue. "This team plays better than any DePaul team I have seen in the last five years," stated Purdue coach Gene Keady. "It'll be a Merry Christmas for us now," Coach Ray said.

Christmas 1983

Dear Ray and The Meyer Family:

Please accept our heartfelt best wishes for a very Merry Christmas and a new year that is filled with inner peace. May the Almighty fill your individual and collective cups with love, an abundance of good health, a long, meaningful life, and the happiness of accomplishment born of application of principle to work for God who so thoroughly affects all our lives. May He bless your economic efforts with success for 1984 (the magic Orwell year) and make it a good year for you, Coach, and Tom (Joey's brother) and Joey who begin new lives in new circumstances. God bless you all and may your acceptance of His benefits inspire you to try harder, do more, go further, and enjoy TOTALLY his goodness and your efforts.

> Warmest regards,
> Norm Kozak
> Nathan Yellen

January 2, 1984

Coach Ray Meyer
DePaul University
Chicago, Illinois

Dear Coach Ray:

We hope that you had a pleasant Holiday Season and are now fortified for the 1984 portion of the season. It seems impossible that 1984 is now here with all the unsavory meanings that the Orwell book conjures up. Surely, much of what was feared in that book is on its way to complete fulfillment, and much worse lies in store. But with all of that, do we fall on the ground in despair? Most assuredly not! We are put on earth to Do and for Good. That combination gives us hope, and strength of purpose and power to do.

We spent yesterday afternoon (Rose Bowl) watching Illinois (10-1) getting destroyed by UCLA (6-4-1), seeing the old lesson taught anew—the awesome, seemingly unstoppable forces destroyed by a seemingly lesser force. The Illinois loss was similar to the failure of the potent White Sox offense in the playoffs against Baltimore! The Illinois team used "dark room imagery" (see our Oct. 16, 1983, note); the Sox took to "winning ugly", and in the face of class teams that dug down deep for meaning, they both failed in the clutch. Neither team was able to win on the basis of its strength. Illinois and the Sox joined the list of casualties whose faith was narrow-minded, misplaced. Sad. Somewhere in all of this is a practical lesson for all of us! I wonder if Georgetown would not profit by their examples, too.

We are most interested in your views on the *Power For Living* book that we gave you early in December, in the hope that you would find it useful to the team. Please let us know your opinion of it. Within the past few weeks it seems as if everywhere one turns that book is being publicized, and by so many different people. We were present at the Biscayne game and watched you leap out of your seat in happiness over Jack Lattner's drive-in lay-up. It was a sight and good feeling!

So, have a good and successful Western road trip and do well! Take Pepperdine out fast and keep them out; they really are not that good, and St. Mary's isn't either; certainly neither are real matches for DePaul.

You must consciously avoid the haughty spirit that Georgetown has seemingly succumbed to in recent weeks. Their game is different since they played DePaul, and though they are winning, it seems that "Ewing (Patrick) & Company" are not doing it like they were at the beginning of the season. They seem to be in a crisis, great though they are, and how will they face it? Will they examine themselves to find the basis for correcting their condition? Tough time, but they must find themselves as Illinois and the Sox must, as well. Ultimately, holistic or synergic behavior is all that works permanently, for it is all that looks to positive substance and God. Fads and "winning ugly" are only temporary, inadequate contrivances for "doing under control". Let Us hear from you. God Love You all.

Your friends,
Norm and Nate

January 10, 1984

Ray Meyer, Coach
DePaul University
1011 West Belden Avenue
Chicago, Illinois 60614

Dear Ray:

The season moves on well and time with it. It has been for us, as you well know by your comments, a pleasure to be of assistance to you, the kids, and the team over this past 21 months that you and we have been talking about the positive value of a holistic/synergic sports program and its great affect upon life itself. You have encouraged us by your considered comments and examples of the benefits to be achieved, and we look forward to our continued assistance to you and the team and the further growth of our friendship.

During this same time we found that this holistic/synergic program has vast possibilities in so many different areas. Suffice it to say that the need is great for holistic and synergic applications to work, sports, life, etc. It could never have flowered if no practical use could be found, and you provided the impetus for our pursuing the concept further. We are grateful for your kindness, assistance, and friendship.

Last summer we wrote to a few baseball teams who

obviously could use help in their player-program in motivation and the Seattle Mariners sounded interested, but as is so clear: we have no "credentials", though we know our program will work. We have no "endorsers", though Norm and I have enriched our lives because of what we know and will continue to grow. In a world so obsessed with tangible factors, faith has taken a back seat and because someone did not think of such a valuable aid, it does not exist or will not work! This, of course, is foolishness—but it is the way people think!

You, however, know better and have seen as well as known the tangible benefits of our program that creates greater totals than the individual parts and inspires movement under control. We, therefore, ask you as a friend to draw a letter to us of suitable character indicating in forthright, truthful, and honest terms what holism/synergy has done for the team, you, and the kids in order to aid us in bringing those benefits to others, such as Seattle, who are surely in need of them. We have tried to convey these thoughts to you recently, but your schedule has been difficult at best; however, you must know how important this is and how much you are a part of it as well as a true and good friend!

Please write us for there is much other talk that we must share of weighty character also! Thank you as always for your consideration of this note, dear friend. God love you as always.

Norm and Nate

Seattle Mariners

July 19, 1983

Mr. Nathan Yellen
Mr. Norman Kozak
5306 W. Devon Avenue
Chicago, IL 60656

Gentlemen:

Thank you for your proposal concerning holistic baseball. As you may know, we are currently in the midst of a transition and do not anticipate involving ourselves in any new programs in the immediate future. It might be wise to contact Mr. Argyros sometime after the first of the year. The time might be right in 1984.

Kindest regards and best wishes.

Sincerely,

Daniel F. O'Brien
President

January 13, 1984

Dear Ray:

I hope that the kids recover from their various and assort-
ed maladies. It sure seems to us that they get an inordinate
amount of flu and cold-related illnesses. They ought to be on
a balanced vitamin program and getting rest that is more than
just sleep—just a thought.

I (Nate) watched (TV) Villanova upset Georgetown. G-
Town is awesome and I respect them greatly, but they are not
really doing the job, not like the son of a preacher, Waymon
Tisdale, and Oklahoma! THAT is a team and their drive is
beyond BELIEF! I sure would like to see them and the Illinois
team against your kids. Note how the Illinois players fell apart
again against Indiana. They should have destroyed Indiana,
but one first has to get past Bobby Knight (Indiana coach); no
small task! Also, Illinois has a penchant for clutch-failure.

Sorry for the run-off. There is so much more great B-Ball
at the college level nowadays. It's like the style of ball that I
loved watching during my high school days: run and gun
with no quitting. Do well against UAB (Alabama-
Birmingham) tomorrow—break those guys early if the kids
are physically well, and KEEP UAB out of it!

God Love All of You,
Norm and Nate

January 15, 1984

Dear Ray:

Congratulations, you certainly lowered the boom (98-63) and delivered the UAB K.O. punch early as Norm suggested in the December 14 letter!

"Breaking them early and keeping them broken" took on a new dimension with the UAB game. It is this concept that Norm and I so completely believe in that is the basis of the "FEAR" that every team that comes up against DePaul feels. They come in unnerved and if you give them half a chance to recover, they will go after us. Controlled intensity (of will) is the answer when you are under control, as you have said with Kenny P; you are on your way!

This was not a win; it was a VICTORY. I think Al McGuire (Division I TV commentator on NCAA men's basketball and former coach of Marquette University) said this or something like it: "A class team does not play its opponent, if the opponent is bad; the class team plays the ball and avoids the sloppiness." This is what you and the team did Saturday. I hope this is the end of the cliffhangers in which the team "allows" an opposing one to get back into the game!

The momentous occurrences continue to mount: The holistic Ohio and Georgetown games and now the total destruction of a good team (14-3 after yesterday's loss), and keeping them broken!

Most important, in the second half of this season: don't allow the "inner enemy", false pride, to become a factor; nip it in the bud and keep it out of the DePaul Basketball Program. Continue to pursue your "peak performance" level, and with "healthy pride" all will yet be well. This will cause your opponents to remain unnerved while DePaul is under control! The kids are really performing as a "team" in spite of their ailments. God Love You and the Team.

Norm and Nate

Ray Meyer and Gene Bartow (Alabama-Birmington coach) quoted in Chicago *Sun-Times* (1/15/84) article by Joel Bierig:

DePaul climbs all over UAB

This is the best DePaul team of 'em all...
The players are all compatible. They seem to like one another. And it looks like they are trying to do something for the coach in his last year.

GENE BARTOW

Our team is more together than any I've had at DePaul...
I'm closer to this team than any I've had. I think the players want to play for me and are doing the best job they can.

RAY MEYER

On February 1, 1984, both in the AP (Associated Press) WRITERS' Poll and the UPI (United Press International) COACHES' Poll, DePaul was ranked second in the nation. They had upped their record to 16-0 with a victory over UCLA at UCLA by the score of 84-68. Just once before in their history had the Bruins suffered a worse loss at home (Pauley Pavilion). Only first-ranked North Carolina had a better record than the Demons: 17-0. In comparison with last season when DePaul won 21 and lost 12, now they were averaging nearly five points more per game and allowing their opponents two points less. Still, Coach was not entirely happy with the team's defensive play. "We may not be that great individually, but collectively we get the job done," Coach admitted regarding the defense. Maybe, in his own words, this was Coach's way of saying "the whole (defense) is more than the sum of its parts." In any event, Coach was looking ahead to the next three games which he termed "crucial" (St. John's, St. Joseph's, and his alma mater, Notre Dame). "If we can win two of three, we'll be happy. You can't be a hog," he stated.

February, 2, 1984

Dear Coach:

It has been a while since we've written due to Norm being out of town and me with my January tax madness, but you know, as always, that you and the team are on our minds. Specifically, the UCLA game that everyone but Norm and I misread: We were looking for a blow-out EVEN ON THEIR FLOOR because of the "take them out and keep them out" theory from UAB. The team, as you say, has matured and is now the "teamy" team that it takes to do the job and still improving! This is the crunch of the season and you plus the peak performance team are ready for it. As you say, they're together as a team; they love one another and you, as you love them! That is, as we've said so many times—The Key— together with love and controlled intensity (of will) to do the job completely!

In this, your final active season, you have risen above the legend you already are to become something greater. You reached out at the age of 70 to embrace new ideas and pro- grams to achieve positively even greater heights and goals because of your vision and uncompromising search for team, individual, and personal excellence. You are 70 years young and growing; under control and crowing about real teams- manship devoted to holistic purposes and showing how to get it done! It is an honor to call you friend, for you, with your vision and comments, made our advances in holistic/synergic programs possible, and we shall ever be indebted to you for it. It is altogether fitting, because of you, that DePaul should have become the birthplace of Holistic Basketball! Your openness and goodness encouraged us!

Teamsmanship became "teamy"—and the RULE! Under control replaced out of control! The 150 percent effort is becoming possible and you did it, Coach; you did it. This is the real legacy that you will leave: Winning became obsolete when you discovered VICTORY! The future of basketball will never be the same when these principles become the RULE; LIFE will change too, as yours did, and you were there when it all began! We have enjoyed watching it develop and hope for even more before this year draws to a close. Nineteen eighty-four can be upbeat and LIFE GIVING, not as Orwell saw it. These principles are positive and illuminating. They replace negativism and show the way rather than remaining in darkness. Thanks.

The 1983-84 season has shown yet another facet of Ray Meyer: the man who adapts to new conditions with thought and action. Your approach and action are somewhat changed, yet the mark of you is on these kids and the odyssey moves on. It seems to us that you have affected this team more than you have impacted on any other group of kids in the past, and the feeling of the "sixth man" is becoming noticeable when the kids are playing—home and away! God grant that it endures and grows stronger. The prescription for healthy pride is still: one game at a time, control of self, and teaminess with love.

With trust in God and peak performance under control, all will yet be well. Warm regards to you, the team, and coaches. God love and protect all of you.

Norm and Nate

DePaul wasn't hoggish! Of the aforementioned three "crucial" games that Coach said the Demons would be happy to win two, that's just what they did! Sandwiched between DePaul's overtime "gift" win over St. John's (59-57) and their "sweet" win over Notre Dame (62-54) was a 58-45 loss to St. Joseph's, the team that eliminated them in the opening game of the 1981 NCAA Tournament. Coach had predicted that his team would lose this game. "We came in here (Palestra) so confident and relaxed, but I knew we weren't going to play well," he uttered.

Some may say that this game was a defeat for the holistic approach. Contrariwise, it was a VICTORY! DePaul fell victim to the "backslide of false pride", the same enemy Georgetown succumbed to. We had forewarned Coach in our January 15 letter to nip "false pride" in the bud. Power of will and false pride work against each other. As one "goes up", the other "goes down", and vice versa.

March 3, 1984

Dear Ray:

In these final moments before the Tournament we want to share these thoughts with you. When Norm and I seized upon the concept of Number 7, namely, 700 wins, 70 years of age, and 7 seasons of great basketball, from the 1977-78 Club of Norwood (Ron)/Garland (Gary) to the 1983-84 TEAM, we never really envisioned this final year of the seven. This year is the ONE of all the seven, for it is the first TRUE TEAM that we have seen. You have brought holism to this TEAM and created a condition that now awaits your final handling—ALL THE WAY IN THE NCAA! No Final Four goals anymore—all the way! Play "as if" you're No. 1 and you will BECOME No. 1! But you must do it—positively!

A lot has passed between us in almost two years and we would not have traded the shared experience for the world, but now you have to take all the essential steps to see that the best players are playing their best on the floor at ALL times. You must be positive in all comments from here on, as far as the kids are concerned, in the media. It should be "My 11 starters" positively. As ever, Norm and I are available to talk with you, but specifically, WE CAN HELP with INSPIRITING Patterson (Kenny), Embry (Marty), et al. Our only purpose is to help your players to win the "inner game" within themselves, so they can get everything God put in them, out, at 150 percent effort; combining this with your expertise on the floor and by doing right, you must of NECESSITY—come out on top in the "outer game". After all, with God's help—how can you fail? We saw the movie, didn't we? *Chariots of Fire*! It's all yours: take the reins of the chariot in your hands and let's go ALL THE WAY!

God Love You and the TEAM,
Norm and Nate

March 6, 1984

Coach Ray Meyer
DePaul University
1011 West Belden Avenue
Chicago, Illinois 60614

Dear Ray:

By Saturday night Phase 1 of the 1983-84 season will be over; then comes the Tournament. It is worthy to note (and the kids should know this) that the basketball writers chose (for their All America Team) 10 players from essentially the top 6 teams in America and only one of those teams was not represented—US—DePaul! This TEAM and you have beaten 4 of the top 20 from Louisville to Georgetown and have something none of them has: THE METHOD! Your TEAM has HOLISM and the MOMENTUM to go all the way. This TEAM will have to be BEATEN: It will not lose and being BEATEN is no disgrace, but losing from here on is unacceptable. This TEAM must comport itself as if it is Number 1, for how is it to become Number 1, if it does not play as if it is Number 1.

Wherever they (tournament committee) send DePaul, the TEAM must play the game, not the opponent. These kids have seen it all by now, and know what to do. Now they must play under control *all* of the time. No screw-offs, screw-ups, or hot dogging—just first class basketball. This TEAM and you believe in the "teamy" concept and that is what it is ALL about! Peak performances; easy does it; under control with a "teamy" team; take your opponent out early and KEEP HIM OUT OF THE GAME by BLOWOUT! The kids must win the "inner game" so the team can win the "outer game"; practice is now merged into the outer game. Did we miss anything? Oh, yes, as ever, with LOVE and for GOD! If we did miss anything, you'll put it in.

God Love this Whole DePaul TEAM and Protect it so it can do what it must DO. That is all that is needed.

Warmest regards,

Norm and Nate

P.S. Personal to you, Ray,

If at any time in these two years we said anything that hurt you or that seemed out of line, we apologize for the appearance, for no such thing was ever intended! We sought only to help and be positively beneficial by telling the truth lovingly to you, and through you, to the kids. So now, to this ONE season of the final seven—a lifetime of accomplishment in one season; with the holistic tool, you now have another lifetime to look forward to, and look at the legacy that you will leave behind to aid people to grow. It is an honor to know you, Mr. Meyer, as friend, and to have shared our experiences. God Love You.

March 8, 1984

Dear Coach:

With Lemone (Lampley) out with a twisted ankle, Dallas (Comegys) with a bad wrist, Lawrence West with the flu, Tyrone and his pains, Embry and his knees, etc., we're surprised you can field two healthy players for a one-on-one or a game of H O R S E!* For openers, you have Marquette, and in a week or so the NCAA Tournament. You have the only HOLISTIC TEAM in the country and that is everything! Take heart, courage, and FAITH IN THE LORD, for HE IS a tree of LIFE to all who hold HIM fast. In spite of your problems, you and the TEAM will come out on top, with LOVE, DETERMINATION, and WILL.

Love,
Norm and Nate

* Beginning with the letter H, each player is given a letter of H O R S E whenever he fails to duplicate the shot of the player he follows. The player remaining after each of the other players has five letters is the winner.

DePaul finished the regular season with a record of 26 wins and 2 losses. After the loss to St. Joseph's they also lost to Dayton, but in a rematch four days later they trounced the Flyers by 20 points. The game against Marquette at home (Rosemont Horizon) was the last regular season game ever, as coach, for Coach, on a day, he said, which would be remembered by him for as long as he lived. Seventeen thousand, five hundred and fifty-nine overzealous fans came to pay tribute to Coach and the Meyer family, and he thanked each and every one of them who came to honor him and his family. "Let's get on with the ball game," he pleaded, in an effort to tone down the pre-game applause and festivities.

Marquette scored 13 of the first 15 points to start the second half, but DePaul still won by 15 points, 64-49. After being handed a scissors, Coach was supported by his players as he jubilantly cut the net down, something he had never done before either as player or coach. A celebration party followed.

March 13, 1984

Coach Ray Meyer
DePaul University
1011 West Belden
Chicago, Illinois 60614

Dear Coach:

Well here it is again: NCAA, but for the last time. Exciting, but this time — UNDER CONTROL! You've had a terrific season rising above problems and creating a TEAM that will be remembered forever, because as you have said, "it believes in itself." We know what that can do, if self-control is exercised! Please reread the March 26, 1983, and March 6, 1984, letters: The rules never change — Method is EVERY-THING! Your enemy is still the same one that was there in 1942 (Ray's first year of coaching at DePaul: "false pride"). Take the opposition out EARLY with "healthy pride" in accomplishment, under control to DO as well as you possibly can, and KEEP THEM OUT OF IT PERMANENTLY! Let everyone know that DePaul will have to be positively BEAT-EN, for DePaul will not lose! Believe it and work for it and it will be! VICTORY or a REAL BEATING (with holism-synergy), but no "losing".

Well, that's it; do well and God bless your efforts with

success. God Love You, the Coaches, and the TEAM!

> We Are DePaul,
> Norm and Nate

The memory of three consecutive opening NCAA tourney setbacks lingered on. Here was Coach's final chance to make amends. The "first game stigma" was a monkey on his back. The last thing he wanted was to begin retirement and leave a legacy of "four of those things". For openers, DePaul was paired with Illinois State. Now, it seemed our words of warning about the team becoming too prideful struck home. "In the past, we were overconfident most of the time. This team is quietly confident," Coach declared. Many said DePaul would "choke", but that rap against the team was quickly put to rest. This time the Demons broke the first game hex and advanced to the second round by convincingly beating ISU 75-61. Coach sounded like a criminal who just found out he got a stay of execution. "I've just been reprieved. I have another week," was his response.

Nate wrote Ray a jingle that went like this:

Illinois State was number one, the fun has just begun;
Wake Forest, number two—you know what to do
This game is more than push and shove
It's determined will, controlled performance and love.

The win over ISU was a double victory. DePaul won the "inner game", as well as the outer.

Now it was on to St. Louis for the semifinals of the NCAA's Midwest Regional. The big question: Would Coach be re-reprieved or would Wake Forest prove to be an insurmountable stumbling block on the way to the Final Four? Answer: The reprieves had come to an end. Wake Forest upset DePaul 73-71 in overtime, a game DePaul should have won in regulation time.

The late Bill Veeck, when he was owner of the Chicago White Sox, once said that the nice thing about being a child is that your dreams aren't punctured by harsh reality. With stark reality staring Coach in the face, the look on his face said it all. But the distinction between life and winning must have been clear in his mind. Many have remarked, "there's more to life than winning," and Larry Bird said it best of all: "It's a game. Nobody dies." Moreover, in a crisis situation a man's character shows itself unmistakably.

Coach kept his perspective and maintained his poise. He walked over to the winning coach to shake his hand and offer him his congratulations. He patiently waited for the commercials to end before being interviewed, and when he spoke into the microphone he gave his assessment of the game, but uppermost in his mind was the welfare of his players. He was eager to return to them. He expressed his gratitude and assured them of his love and helpfulness when he saw them. He urged them to walk tall. It was his players he was sorry for, not himself. People would feel sorry for him, but he didn't want them to.

Even though the loss was no joke, he joked. "I'm going to be a fund-raiser now. I can do more for the players that way than I did as a coach." Winston Churchill spoke of life as being a test—and Coach had passed with flying colors! Coach's career-ending game was a repetition of them all—first-class all the way!

March 31, 1984

Norm:

The agony of Wake Forest is over. You ask me how I assess two years with Ray and I say this: You and I saw the birth of HOLISTIC B-ball. Ray was its daddy and we were his constant encouragement! He did it all the way, though I wish I knew entirely WHAT! We saw a 70-year-old man rise again to the occasion and change for the better! The legacy of this TEAM is that he created it; not in his image as he saw life, but in ours, and he loved every minute of it! God love him. We are his friends and we have done it as no one ever has before. It was and it is everything. We did it with chutzpah (nerve) and love and he, by listening and performance.

No doubt I wish some things were done differently, like St. Joe's and Dayton explained—but who but God is perfect? We have no recriminations on what we said or did. We were there and we helped it happen. No one can ever take that from us!

By the way, God love you, too! Thanks for "dreying my kop with your mishegoss!"*

Nate

* turning my head with your craziness—craziness from the standpoint of nonbelievers.

April 1, 1984

Nate:

It's been said that "A mind stretched by a new idea never regains its former size." As for the Blue Demons, although they unconsciously absorbed holism, their minds were never chock-full of it—permanently s-t-r-e-t-c-h-e-d.

Regardless of the outcome of the Wake Forest game, you must not overlook that even though Ray had 42 years of coaching experience, he was still a "holistic rookie", with no beaten path to follow. He is to be extolled for his courage, for he didn't flinch from applying TRUTH (the focal point of his life) as he interpreted it.

Norm

April 2, 1984

Dear Ray:

John Thompson (coach of Georgetown, NCAA champion) was interviewed after the Final Four game and credited his team's victory (Cable News Network) to a lesson he learned this season. It is to protect against giving an opposing team a chance to get back into the game when it is down and nearly out. He learned that lesson at the Horizon on December 10, 1983, from DePaul—a team that not only would not quit, but was VICTORIOUS.

This is the testimonial to this 1983-84 season: You developed a TRUE TEAM, a "TEAMY" one that did more than defeat Georgetown; it rose above illness and injury, setback and problems, to prove that even without stars—a TEAM can DO! And this team (plus you) DID!

We wish you and your loved ones a Happy Easter. Call us when you return from your trip.* Bon Voyage and

      Warm regards,

      Nate

* In a speech delivered by Coach at a post-tournament luncheon at Alumni Hall, commemorating his 42 years of coaching and loyalty to DePaul (everyone who attended was given a plaque of him in which his autograph was inscribed), he

repeated with tongue in cheek an opinion which someone offered him after his final game with Wake Forest: God simply had not chosen DePaul in the pool!

Coach and Mrs. Meyer were going on an extended trip, during which they would visit Rome and meet His Holiness, the Pope. We wished them well.

4
EPILOGUE: RETIREMENT?

Coach had retired from coaching but not from active, creative living. At Three Lakes, Wisconsin, he would continue on with his Summer Basketball Camp; and at the university, as assistant to the athletic director (Ed Manetta), he would help raise funds. Previously he had accepted WGN's radio offer to do color commentary for the '84-85 season; writing a book was also a consideration.

When we visited him at Alumni Hall, he talked of these things and on all sports in general. To Coach, money is not all-important. He would rather do something that he would be happy at, rather than something more lucrative but not personally satisfying. God and his family are and always will be his "top priorities"; his continuous love and concern for the well-being of his players (past and present) is no less an extension of himself. When his players experienced good fortune he was overjoyed, and when they had reversals, the bells tolled for him. He took their reversals personally.

Coach is a humble man. Although he is in the Hall of

Fame, the Hall of Fame is not in him. He never spoke of his accomplishments, but every game he coached is forever etched in his memory.

Ultimately he would by-line a regular article for the *Chicago Sun-Times*, and have a weekly Sunday TV show (The Ray Meyer Show).

November 13, 1984

Dear Ray:

I was greeted today with the news that in a pre-season AP Basketball Poll for the 1984-85 season, DePaul is third-ranked nationally, and I felt good about it. There are not many better, if they do their job, than that TEAM of yours. Once again, the fall ritual of writing you and wishing all well. This year you get to see the machine that you created, instead of pushing the button to get it moving. You gave it life, direction, goal, meaning, purpose, and METHOD with which to do its job—that "TEAMY" TEAM of yours that you turned over to Joey. Most assuredly, your work with those kids using the holistic/synergic method and the power of you created this very situation. No father ever gave his son a better opportunity to do his job that included a TEAM like this! You and the method's principles live on and Joey can take it the rest of the way.

Of course, staying under control and playing "as if" the TEAM is Number 1 is everything, and Joey will have to hold on; but look what he has to hold on to! This is your handiwork and you must be silently proud, for this is positively the work of your mind, heart, and hands—for God. You are the father of Holistic Basketball and now, hopefully, your product will go on.

Happy 1984-85 season, COACH. God Love You, the TEAM, coaches, and your loved ones.

Warm regards,
Nate

November 14, 1984

Dear Ray:

With all the established stars of prior years gone, and the assurance that you had a few "take charge" players around to "pull it out" in "game" situations a thing of the past, you faced the '83-84 season with a young team that although talented, had a distance to go. Your approach was to create a "teamy" team whereby the good of the player and the good of the team would be identical and mutually reinforcing.

QUESTION:

To what extent do you believe that a holistic attitude and state of mind fosters peak experiences and performances creating such a "teamy" TEAM?

Norm

DePaul University

Department of Athletics   1011 West Belden Avenue   312/321-8010
                                  Chicago, IL 60614

Dear Norm,

In creating a team you must get the players to play together as a unit. You operate on the theory that the hand is the sum total of the fingers. They act and perform together. Holism is the sum total of all of the team's players.

I generally tried to develop a team by getting to know the players. My approach to them was to treat them individually with the concept of a team in mind. For example, I knew Patterson was the playmaker and he was instructed to handle the ball and be creative and show initiative. He was a scorer in high school and I convinced him that he was more valuable to the team as a playmaker.

Jerry McMillan was the shooter. I wanted him to shoot when he was set. He was not to force a shot or take a hurried shot, but he was to wait for the opportunity.

Marty Embry was the center. He was the strong man in the middle. His job was not scoring but to defend against the big man and to rebound. That would be his greatest contribution and if an easy shot was available, he was to take it.

Kevin Holmes was the power forward. He had to score a little, hit the short jumper but concentrate on getting his scoring under or in close to the basket. Above all, he had to rebound.

Tyrone Corbin was the small forward. He was to depend on his quickness. He was supposed to take his shots from the floor; go down on a fast break and sneak in for the offensive boards. He had to be able to handle the ball against the press and be able to dribble the ball if need be. He was the outlet pass against pressure defenses whenever the guards were in trouble. Ty had to do many things to make the team go. It was important that he be able to handle quick forwards or big forwards.

Dallas Comergys was instant offense. He had problems on defense but he was a real threat on offense and an exceptional rebounder. He had to be convinced of his shot selection. We did not want him to force long turnaround jumpers. When he did this he hurt the team.

Tony Jackson was another offensive player. He usually replaced McMillan. We did not want him to do what Mac did; we wanted him to penetrate and get shots on the move. One was a set shooter and the other was a better shooter on the move.

The whole idea was to give each player a role and let him fulfill it. We always stressed that the team wins and the team loses.

On defense, the emphasis was always on team defense. If one player was beaten, someone was to help. We had a strong side, the side the ball was on, and we had a weak side opposite the ball. Our theory was that if a basket was scored on our man, it was scored on our whole team, not just one individual.

On offense, one player can't score by himself. He needs help. The way to help one another is by movement—movement of the players and the ball. This creates opportunities. We had a few this past season and we capitalized on them, generally. This team knew its job and did it!

Yours,
Ray Meyer

November 25, 1984

Dear Ray:

Thanks for your letter expressing your holistic viewpoints as related to the 1983-84 "teamy" TEAM, at this hectic time for you. Considering Thanksgiving, your Sun-Times column, regular Sunday TV show, and broadcasting of Blue Demon games with Joe McConnell, it shows real character on your behalf.

Ray, at the end of the road to Lexington,* when hopefully, God has "chosen DePaul in the pool," I'd like the opportunity to explain to you the HOLISTIC approach in sports and its ramifications in depth. I think you'll find it illuminating, enlightening, and inspiriting.

I feel, given basic skills and talent, ANY team with the "know-how" of tapping and utilizing this relatively untapped resource, making space and factoring in this "weapon" as a regular part of its arsenal, has got to come out on top. For God is TRUTH and TRUTH is the "club" that knocks down opposition.

God bless you and your loved ones, good health, and I hope that you're enjoying your new role in sports.

Warm regards,

Norm

---

* Lexington, Kentucky, the site of the 1985 NCAA finals.

The Beginning...
of Holism in Everything
It's about time you LIVE it! You'll LOVE it!

ABOUT THE AUTHORS

Norman Kozak was born in Chicago, Illinois. He graduated from the University of Illinois and holds a bachelor's degree in journalism. Mr. Kozak is a salesman and an avid reader with a long-standing interest in the holistic approach to sport and life. His poem, "A Bit of Wisdom", was published by the national Library of Poetry in 1998 as part of a collection entitled *A Painted Garden*.

Nathan Yellen graduated from DePaul University with a degree in accounting. Currently, he utilizes holistic principles in his career as a practicing CPA. He has also done historical research in Spain on Christopher Columbus. Mr. Yellen is married and has two children.

GLOSSARY

DEFEAT: Holistic losing; not just "losing".

HOLISTIC: Pertaining to the whole person—body, mind, and spirit. "The whole is greater than the sum of its parts," is the main principle of the holistic approach.

PEAK
EXPERIENCE: Channeling of holistic energies and powers whereby the whole of behavior becomes more than the sum of its parts.

SPIRIT: The fundamental life force; Divine Energy of Truth and Love; in a nonreligious sense, the dimension of meaning and purpose.

SCHLEP: An inept team; a player whose performance is "less than the sum of his parts."

SYNERGY: Godly holism—the uniting of the individual will with the Divine Will; parts working together in the service of a common goal, each enhancing and increasing the effectiveness of the others.

VICTORY: Holistic winning; not just "winning".

WILL: The choosing, striving, and achieving faculty.

BIBLIOGRAPHY

Arieti, S. *The Will to Be Human*. Quadrangle Books, Inc., 1972.

Assagioli, R. *The Act of Will*. Penguin Books Inc., 1976.

Colbert, J. *Golf Magazine*, June 1975, as quoted in L.R. Keck, *The Spirit of Synergy: God's Power and You*. Abingdon Nashville, 1978.

Dyer, Dr. W.W. *Real Magic: Creating Miracles in Everyday Life*. New York: Harper Collins, 1992.

Freeman, A.M. & DeWolf, R. *The 10 Dumbest Mistakes Smart People Make and How to Avoid Them: Simple and Sure Techniques for Gaining Control of Your Life*. New York: Harper Collins, 1992.

Goble, F. *Beyond Failure: How to Cure a Neurotic Society*. Caroline House Books/Green Hill Publishers, Inc., 1977.

Greenwald, Dr. H. & Rich, E. *The Happy Person*. New York: Stein & Day, 1984.

Henning, J. *Holistic Running*. Atheneum, 1978.

Heschel, A.J. *Maimonides*. Joachim Neugroschel, Tr. Farrar, Straus &Giroux, 1955.

Hordern, W. *A Layman's Guide to Protestant Theology*. New York: Macmillan, 1955.

Jaffee, D.T. *Healing from Within*. New York: Alfred A. Knopf, 1980.

James, W. *The Principles of Psychology*, Vol. 2. New York: Dover Publications, 1950.

Keck, L.R. *The Spirit of Synergy: God's Power and You.*. Abingdon Nashville, 1978.

Loehr, J.E. *The New Toughness Training for Sports: Mental, Emotional, and Physical Conditioning from One of the World's Premier Sports Psychologists.* New York: Dutton, 1994.

Maslow, A.H. "Some Educational Implications of the Humanistic Psychologies," *Harvard Educational Review*, Fall, 1968, as quoted in Frank Goble, *Beyond Failure: How to Cure a Neurotic Society.* Caroline House Books/Green Hill Publishers, Inc., 1977.

May, R. *Love and Will*. New York: Dell Publishing Co., Inc., 1969.

Mays, C. *A Strategy for Winning...in Business, in Sports, in Family, in Life.* New York: Lincoln-Bradley, 1991.

Montante, J.C. *Life...A Competitive Nightmare: How to Target Yourself for Success.* Apex Books, 1991.

Nideffer, R.M., Ph.D. *The Inner Athlete: Mind Plus Muscle for Winning.* New York: Thomas Y. Crowell Company, 1976.

Otto, H.A. *Love Today: A New Exploration.* New York: Association Press, 1972.

Plimpton, G. *The X Factor: A Quest for Excellence.* W.W. Norton, 1995.

Robbins, A. & McClendon III, J. *Unlimited Power: A Black Choice.* New York: Simon & Schuster, 1997.

Sheen, F. D.D. *Life is Worth Living.* McGraw-Hill Inc., 1953.

Shostrom, E.L. *Actualizing Therapy: Foundations for a Scientific Ethic.* San Diego: Edits, 1976.

Smuts, J.C. *Holism and Evolution.* New York: Macmillan, 1926.

Stein, M. *Practicing Wholeness: Analytical Psychology and Jungian Thought.* New York: Continuum, 1996.

Sutherland, N.S. *The International Dictionary of Psychology.* New York: Continuum, 1996.

Taylor, K.N. *The Living Bible*, paraphrased: Holman Illustrated Ed, A.J. Holman Co., 1973.

Tillich, P. *The Courage to Be.* Yale University Press, 1952.

Werner, H.D. *Cognitive Therapy: A Humanistic Approach.* Free Press, 1982.

Wittig, A.F. Ph.D. *Schaum's Outline of Theory and Problems of Introduction to Psychology.* McGraw-Hill Inc., 1977.